BLUEPRINTS IN PSYCHIATRY

Blueprints: USMLE Steps 2 & 3 Review Series

General Series Editor:

Bradley S. Marino, M.D., M.P.P.
Department of Pediatrics
Johns Hopkins Hospital
Baltimore, Maryland

CURRENT BOOKS IN THE SERIES:

Blueprints in Medicine
Blueprints in Obstetrics and Gynecology
Blueprints in Pediatrics
Blueprints in Surgery

BLUEPRINTS IN

PSYCHIATRY

Michael J. Murphy, MD, MPH
Clinical Fellow in Psychiatry
Harvard Medical School
Boston, Massachusetts
Resident in Adult Psychiatry
McLean Hospital
Belmont, Massachusetts

Ronald L. Cowan, MD, PhD
Clinical Fellow in Psychiatry
Harvard Medical School
Boston, Massachusetts
Resident in Adult Psychiatry
McLean Hospital
Belmont, Massachusetts

Faculty Advisor:
Lloyd I. Sederer, MD
Associate Professor of Clinical Psychiatry
Harvard Medical School
Boston, Massachusetts
Medical Director
McLean Hospital
Belmont, Massachusetts

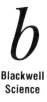

**Blackwell
Science**

Blackwell Science
Editorial Offices:
350 Main Street, Malden, Massachusetts 02148, USA
Osney Mead, Oxford OX2 0EL, England
25 John Street, London WC1N 2BL, England
23 Ainslie Place, Edinburgh EH3 6AJ, Scotland
54 University Street, Carlton, Victoria 3053, Australia

Other Editorial Offices:
Blackwell Wissenschafts-Verlag GmbH Kurfürstendamm 57, 10707 Berlin, Germany
Blackwell Science KK, MG Kodenmacho Nihombashi
   Chuo-ku Tokyo 104, Japan

Distributors:
USA
   Blackwell Science, Inc.
   Commerce Place
   350 Main Street
   Malden, Massachusetts 02148
   (Telephone orders: 800-215-1000
   or 781-388-8250; Fax orders: 781-388-8270)
Canada
   Login Brothers Book Company
   324 Saulteaux Crescent
   Winnipeg, Manitoba
   Canada, R3J 3T2
   (Telephone orders: 204-224-4068)

Australia
   Blackwell Science Pty., Ltd.
   54 University Street
   Carlton, Victoria 3053
   (Telephone orders: 03-9347-0300;
   Fax orders: 03-9349-3016)
Outside North America and Australia
   Blackwell Science, Ltd.
   c/o Marston Book Services, Ltd.
   P.O. Box 269, Abingdon
   Oxon OX14 4YN
   England
   (Telephone orders: 44-01235-465500;
   Fax orders: 44-01235-465555)

Acquisitions: Joy Ferris Denomme
Production: Karen Feeney
Manufacturing: Lisa Flanagan
Typeset by Publication Services
Printed and bound by Capital City Press
©1998 by Blackwell Science, Inc.
Printed in the United States of America

98 99 00 5 4 3 2

Library of Congress Cataloging-in-Publication Data
Murphy, Michael, 1966—
     Blueprints in psychiatry / Michael Murphy, Ronald Cowan ; faculty advisor,
Lloyd Sederer.
        p.   cm.—(Blueprints)
     Includes bibliographical references and index.
     ISBN 0-86542-503-5 (pb)
     1. Psychiatry—Outlines, syllabi, etc. I. Cowan, Ronald.
II. Sederer, Lloyd I. III. Title. IV. Series: The blueprints series.
     [DNLM: 1. Mental Disorders—examination questions.
2. Psychotropic Drugs—examination questions.   WM 18.2 M978b 1997]
RC457.2.M87   1997
616.89'0076—dc21
DNLM/DLC
for Library of Congress   97-7347
                                                                   CIP

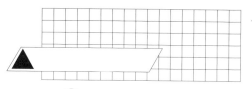

Contents

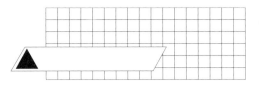

Preface

Fourth-year medical students, interns, and residents are chronically sleep deprived, have little time to study due to their clinical duties, and have a low tolerance for medical literature that is not clear and to the point. All too often as a medical student, and now as a resident, I have heard my colleagues bemoan the fact that there is no succinct, clinical text on each of the core subjects tested on the USMLE Steps 2 & 3. These trainees need review materials they can digest quickly, perhaps a subject in a weekend, which will enable them to answer correctly the majority of questions in each discipline. This attitude is especially evident for the USMLE Step 3, for example, where surgical residents are tested on pediatrics although they have not completed a clinical rotation in the discipline for two years.

Our goal in writing *Blueprints in Psychiatry* was to enable the reader to review the core material quickly and efficiently. The topics were chosen after analyzing over 2,000 review questions, which we believed were representative of the psychiatry questions on the USMLE Steps 2 & 3 exams. This book is not meant to be comprehensive, but rather it is composed of the "high-yield" topics that consistently appear on these exams.

The questions on the USMLE Steps 2 & 3 are now crafted into clinical vignettes. To assist you in studying for this new format, the material in this book is presented either as the workup of a symptom or as a discussion of a particular disease or pathological process. Although this series is designed for the medical student or resident reviewing for the USMLE, we believe the books will be equally useful to all medical students during their clerkships or subinternships.

We hope that you find *Blueprints in Psychiatry* informative and useful. We welcome any feedback you may have about this text or any others in the Blueprints series.

Bradley S. Marino, MD, MPP
Blueprints Series Editor
c/o Blackwell Science, Inc.
Commerce Place
350 Main Street
Malden, MA 02148

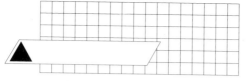

Acknowledgments

We would like to thank the faculty, staff, and residents of the McLean Hospital for their support throughout the writing of this text. We would especially like to thank Dr. Lloyd I. Sederer for patiently guiding us to its completion.

Ronald L. Cowan, M.D., Ph.D.
Michael J. Murphy, M.D., M.P.H.

My thanks to the trainees, staff, and patients of McLean Hospital who have made learning and teaching a pleasure.

Lloyd I. Sederer, MD

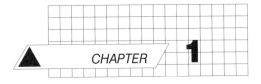
Psychotic Disorders

*P*sychotic disorders are a collection of disorders in which **psychosis** predominates the symptom complex. Psychosis is defined as a gross impairment in reality testing. Specific psychotic symptoms, including delusions, hallucinations, ideas of reference, and disorders of thought, also are present. Table 1-1 classifies the psychotic disorders.

It is important to understand that psychotic disorders are different from mood disorders with psychotic features. Patients can present with a severe episode of depression and have delusions or with a manic episode with delusions and hallucinations. These patients do not have a primary psychotic disorder, rather their psychosis is secondary to a mood disorder.

The diagnoses described below are among the most severely disabling of mental disorders. Disability is in part because of the extreme degree of social and occupational dysfunction associated with these disorders.

▶ SCHIZOPHRENIA

Schizophrenia is a disorder in which patients have psychotic symptoms and social and/or occupational dysfunction that persists for at least 6 months.

Epidemiology

Schizophrenia affects 1% of the population. The typical age of onset is the early 20s for men and the late 20s for women. Women are more likely to have a "first break" later in life; in fact, about one-third of women have an onset of illness after age 30. Schizophrenia is diagnosed disproportionately among the lower socioeconomic classes; although theories exist for this finding, none have been substantiated.

TABLE 1-1

Psychotic Disorders

Schizophrenia	Brief psychotic disorder
Schizophreniform disorder	Shared psychotic disorder
Schizoaffective disorder	Delusional disorder

Etiology

The etiology of schizophrenia is unknown. There is a clear inheritable component, but familial incidence is sporadic and it does occur in families with no history of the disease. Schizophrenia is widely believed to have a neurobiologic basis. The most notable theory is the **dopamine hypothesis**, which posits that schizophreniais due to hyperactivity in brain dopaminergic pathways. This theory is consistent with the efficacy of antipsychotics (which block dopamine receptors) and the ability of drugs (such as cocaine) that stimulate dopaminergic activity to induce psychosis. Postmortem studies also have shown higher levels of dopamine receptors in specific subcortical nuclei of schizophrenics than with normal brains. More recent studies have focused on structural and functional abnormalities through brain imaging of schizophrenics and control populations. No one finding or theory to date is adequate in explaining the etiology and pathogenesis of this complex disease.

Clinical Manifestations

History and Mental Status Examination

Schizophrenia is a disorder characterized by what has been termed **positive** and **negative symptoms,** a pattern of **social and occupational deterioration,** and persistence of the illness for at least **6 months.** Positive symptoms are characterized by the **presence** of unusual thoughts, perceptions, and behaviors (e.g., hallucinations, delusions, agitation); negative symptoms are characterized by the **absence** of normal social and mental functions (e.g., lack of motivation, isolation, anergia). The positive versus negative distinction was made in a nosologic attempt to identify subtypes of schizophrenia and because some medications seem to be more effective in treating negative symptoms. Clinically, patients often exhibit both positive and negative symptoms at the same time. Table 1-2 lists common positive and negative symptoms.

To make the diagnosis, one must meet two (or more) of the following criteria: hallucinations, delusions, disorganized speech, grossly disorganized or catatonic behavior, or negative symptoms. There also

TABLE 1-2
Positive and Negative Symptoms of Schizophrenia

Negative symptoms

Affective flattening	Decreased expression of emotion such as lack of expressive gestures
Alogia	Literally "lack of words," including poverty of speech and of speech content
Asociality	Few friends, activities, interests; impaired intimacy, little sexual interest

Positive symptoms

Hallucinations	Auditory, visual, tactile, and/or olfactory hallucinations; voices that are commenting
Delusions	Often described by content; persecutory, grandiose, paranoid, religious; ideas of reference, thought broadcasting, thought insertion, thought withdrawal
Bizarre behavior	Aggressive/agitated, odd clothing or appearance, odd social behavior, repetitive-stereotyped behavior

Adapted from Andreasen, Introductory Textbook of Psychiatry. American Psychiatric Press. 1995:207.

TABLE 1-1
Subtypes of Schizophrenia

Paranoid	Paranoid delusions, frequent auditory hallucinations, affect *not* flat
Catatonic	Motoric immobility or excessive, purposeless motor activity, maintenance of a rigid posture echolalia
Disorganized	Disorganized speech, disorganized behavior, flat or inappropriate affect. Not catatonic
Undifferentiated (probably most common)	Delusions, hallucinations, disorganized speech, catatonic behavior, negative symptoms. *Criteria not met for paranoid, catatonic, or disorganized*
Residual	Met criteria for schizophrenia, now resolved, i.e., no hallucinations, no prominent delusions, etc., but residual negative symptoms or attenuated delusions, hallucinations, or thought disorder

Adapted from Andreasen, Introductory Textbook of Psychiatry. American Psychiatric Press. 1995:213.

must be social and/or occupational dysfunction. The patient must be ill for at least 6 months.

Patients with schizophrenia generally have a history of abnormal premorbid functioning. The prodrome of schizophrenia includes poor social skills, social withdrawal, and unusual (although not frankly delusional) thinking. Inquiring about the premorbid history may help to distinguish schizophrenia from a psychotic illness secondary to mania or drug ingestion.

Schizophrenics are at high risk for suicide. Approximately one-third will attempt suicide and 10% will complete suicide. Risk factors for suicide include male gender, age <30 years, chronic course, prior depression, and recent hospital discharge.

The *Diagnostic and Statistical Manual of Mental Disorders*, 4th edition (DSM-IV) recognizes five subtypes of schizophrenia: paranoid, disorganized, catatonic, undifferentiated, and residual. The subtypes of schizophrenia are useful as descriptors but have not been shown to be reliable or valid subtypes. Table 1-3 describes these subtypes.

Differential Diagnosis
The differential diagnosis of an acute psychotic episode is broad and challenging (Table 1-4). Once a medical or substance-related condition has been ruled out,

the task is to differentiate schizophrenia from a schizoaffective disorder, a mood disorder with psychotic features, a delusional disorder, or a personality disorder.

Management
Antipsychotic agents are primarily used in treatment. These medications are used to treat acute psychotic episodes and to maintain patients in remission or with chronic illness. Antipsychotic medications are discussed in Chapter 11. **Psychosocial treatments**, including stable reality-oriented psychotherapy, family support, psychoeducation, social and vocational skills training, and attention to details of living situation (housing, roommates, daily activities), are critical to the long-term management of these patients.

Key Points
Schizophrenia

1. Is characterized by psychosis and social/occupational dysfunction;
2. Must last for at least 6 months;
3. Has a 10% suicide rate (30% attempt);
4. Is treated with antipsychotics and psychosocial support.

▶ **SCHIZOAFFECTIVE DISORDER**
Patients with schizoaffective disorder have psychotic episodes that **resemble schizophrenia** bu

with prominent mood disturbances. Their psychotic symptoms, however, must persist for some time in the absence of any mood syndrome.

Epidemiology

Lifetime prevalence is estimated at 0.5% to 0.8%. Age of onset is similar to schizophrenia (late teens to early 20s). Schizoaffective patients are more likely than schizophrenics but less likely than mood-disordered patients to have a remission after treatment.

Etiology

The etiology of schizoaffective disorder is unknown. It may be a variant of schizophrenia, a variant of a mood disorder, a distinct psychotic syndrome, or simply superimposed mood disorder and psychotic disorder.

Clinical Manifestations

History and Mental Status Examination

Patients with schizoaffective disorder have the typical symptoms of schizophrenia and coincidentally a major mood disturbance, such as a manic or depressive episode. They must also have periods of illness in which they have psychotic symptoms **without a major mood disturbance**. Mood disturbances need to be present for a substantial portion of the illness.

There are two subtypes of schizoaffective disorder recognized in the DSM-IV, **depressive** and **bipolar**, that are determined by the nature of the mood-disturbance episodes.

Differential Diagnosis

Mood disorders with psychotic features, such as in mania or psychotic depression, are different from schizoaffective disorder in that these patients have persistence (for at least 2 weeks) of the psychotic symptoms after the mood symptoms have resolved. Schizophrenia is differentiated from schizoaffective disorder by the absence of a prominent mood disorder in the course of the illness.

It is important to distinguish the prominent negative symptoms of the schizophrenic from the **lack of energy** or **anhedonia** in the depressed patient with schizoaffective disorder. More distinct symptoms of a mood disturbance (such as depressed mood and sleep disturbance) should indicate a true coincident mood disturbance.

Management

Patients are treated with medications that target the psychosis and the mood disorder. Typically, these patients require the **combination of an antipsychotic medication and a mood stabilizer**. An antidepressant or electroconvulsive therapy may be needed for an acute depressive episode.

TABLE 1-4

Causes of acute psychotic syndromes

Major psychiatric disorders
  Acute exacerbation of schizophrenia
  Atypical psychoses (e.g., schizophreniform)
  Depression with psychotic features
  Mania
Drug abuse and withdrawal
  Alcohol withdrawal
  Amphetamines and cocaine
  Phencyclidine (PCP) and hallucinogens
  Sedative-hypnotic withdrawal
Prescription drugs
  Anticholinergic agents
  Digitalis toxicity
  Glucocorticoids and adrenocorticotropic hormone (ACTH)
  Isoniazid
  L-Dopa and other dopamine agonists
  Nonsteroidal anti-inflammatory agents
  Withdrawal from MAOIs
Other toxic agents
  Carbon disulfide
  Heavy metals
Neurologic causes
  AIDS encephalopathy
  Brain tumor
  Complex partial seizures
  Early Alzheimer's or Pick's disease
  Huntington's disease
  Hypoxic encephalopathy
  Infectious viral encephalitis
  Lupus cerebritis
  Neurosyphilis
  Stroke
  Wilson's disease
Metabolic causes
  Acute intermittent porphyria
  Cushing's syndrome
  Early hepatic encephalopathy
  Hypo- and hypercalcemia
  Hypoglycemia
  Hypo- and hyperthyroidism
  Paraneoplastic syndromes (limbic encephalitis)
Nutritional causes
  Niacin deficiency (pellagra)
  Thiamine deficiency (Wernicke-Korsakoff syndrome)
  Vitamin B_{12} deficiency

Reproduced with permission from Arana GW, Hyman SE, and Rosenbaum JF, Handbook of Psychiatric Drug Therapy, 3rd Edition. Boston: Little, Brown & Co. 1995:24.

Key Points

In schizoaffective disorder

1. There are mood disturbances *with* psychotic episodes;
2. There are periods of psychosis *without* a mood disturbance;
3. Treatment is with antipsychotics and mood stabilizers.

► SCHIZOPHRENIFORM DISORDER

Essentially, this is schizophrenia that fails to last for 6 months and does not involve social withdrawal.

Epidemiology

The validity of this diagnosis is under question. Outcome studies of this disorder indicate that most patients may go on to develop full-blown **schizophrenia,** whereas others appear to develop a **mood disorder.** The diagnosis of schizophreniform disorder may, however, avoid premature diagnosis of patients with schizophrenia before some other disorder, such as bipolar disorder, manifests itself.

Etiology

At this time, the etiology is unknown. At least one study found similarities in brain structural abnormalities between schizophrenics and those with schizophreniform disorder.

Clinical Manifestations

History and Mental Status Examination

Schizophreniform disorder is essentially **short-course schizophrenia** without the requirement of social withdrawal. Patients with this disorder have what appears to be a "full-blown" episode of schizophrenia, including delusions, hallucinations, disorganized speech, or negative symptoms, but the duration of illness including prodromal, active, and residual phases, is from 1 to 6 months. The diagnosis changes to schizophrenia once the symptoms have extended past 6 months, even if the only symptoms left are residual ones.

Differential Diagnosis

Care must be taken to distinguish schizophreniform disorder from a manic or depressive episode with psychotic features. Other causes of an acute psychosis must be ruled out (substance induced or due to a general medical condition).

Management

The disorder is by definition **self-limited.** When symptoms cause severe impairment, treatment is similar to that for the acute treatment of psychosis in schizophrenia.

Key Points

Schizophreniform disorder

1. Resembles schizophrenia;
2. Resolves completely in less than 6 months;
3. Most often results in either schizophrenia or bipolar disorder;
4. Is self-limited.

► DELUSIONAL DISORDER

Delusional disorder is characterized by nonbizarre delusions without other psychotic symptoms. It is rare, its course is chronic, and treatment is supportive.

Epidemiology

This disorder is rare, with a prevalence of <0.05%. Generally, onset is in middle to late life; it affects women more often than men. Its course is **chronic** and **unremitting.**

Etiology

The etiology is unknown. Often, psychosocial stressors appear to be etiologic, such as in a subtype of delusional disorder known as **migration psychosis.** In migration psychosis, the recently immigrated person develops persecutory delusions. Many patients with delusional disorder have a paranoid character premorbidly. Paranoid personality disorder has been found in families with a patient with delusional disorder.

Clinical Manifestations

History and Mental Status Examination

This disorder is characterized by well-systematized **nonbizarre delusions** about things that could happen in real life (such as being followed, poisoned, infected, loved at a distance, having a disease, being deceived by one's spouse or significant other). The delusions must be present for at least 1 month and, other than the delusion, the patient's social adjustment remains normal.

The patient must not meet criteria for schizophrenia. Any mood disorder must be brief relative to the duration of the illness.

Differential Diagnosis

It is important to rule out other psychiatric or medical illnesses that could have caused the delusions. Thereafter, delusional disorder must be distinguished from major depression with psychotic features, mania, schizophrenia, and paranoid personality.

Management

Trials of antipsychotics are appropriate but are often not effective. The primary treatment is **psychotherapy**, taking care to neither support nor refute the delusion to maintain an **alliance** with the patient. Without such an alliance, most patients fall out of treatment; with an alliance, over time, the patient may relinquish the delusions.

Key Points

Delusional disorder

1. Is characterized by nonbizarre delusions;
2. Is chronic and unremitting;
3. Is treated by making a therapeutic alliance.

▶ BRIEF PSYCHOTIC DISORDER

In brief psychotic disorder, the patient experiences a full psychotic episode that is **short-lived**. It can be temporally related to some stressor or occur postpartum but is also seen **without any apparent antecedent**.

Epidemiology

There is insufficient data available to determine prevalence and sex ratio.

Etiology

Etiology is unknown. However, it seems to be associated with borderline personality disorder and schizotypal personality disorder.

Clinical Manifestations

History and Mental Status Examination

In brief psychotic disorder, the patient develops psychotic symptoms that last for at least 1 day but no more than 1 month, followed by eventual return to premorbid functioning. Patients can exhibit any combination of delusions, hallucinations, disorganized speech, or grossly disorganized behavior. There are three recognized subtypes: **with marked stressors** (formerly known as brief reactive psychosis), **without marked stressors**, and **postpartum**. Patients with the postpartum subtype typically develop symptoms within 1 to 2 weeks after delivery that resolve within 2 to 3 months.

Differential Diagnosis

One must rule out schizophrenia, especially if the disorder worsens or persists for over a month (except for postpartum psychosis, which may last 2 to 3 months). A mood disorder such as mania or depression with psychotic features must be ruled out.

Management

Hospitalization may be necessary to protect the patient. Treatment with neuroleptics is common, although the condition is by definition self-limited and so no specific treatment is required. The containing environment of the hospital milieu may be sufficient to help the patient recover.

Key Points

Brief psychotic disorder

1. Is characterized by typical psychotic symptoms;
2. Is short-lived, lasting from 1 to 30 days;
3. Can be preceded by a stressor or can be postpartum;
4. May occur without an antecedent;
5. Is self-limited.

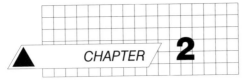

CHAPTER 2

Mood Disorders

*M*ood disorders are among the most common diagnoses in psychiatry. Mood is a persistent emotional state (as differentiated from affect, which is the external display of feelings). There are three major categories of mood disorders according to *The Diagnostic and Statistical Manual of Mental Disorders*, 4th edition: unipolar mood disorders (major depressive disorder, dysthymic disorder), bipolar mood disorders (bipolar I disorder, bipolar II disorder, and cyclothymic disorder), and mood disorders having a known etiology (substance-induced mood disorder and mood disorder due to a general medical condition (Table 2-1).

The best available evidence suggests that mood disorders lie on a continuum with normal mood. Although mania and depression are often viewed as opposite ends of the mood spectrum, they can occur simultaneously in a single individual within a brief period, giving rise to the concept of mixed mood states.

▶ UNIPOLAR DISORDERS

Unipolar disorders are major depressive disorder and dysthymic disorder.

Major Depressive Disorder

Major depressive disorder is diagnosed after a single episode of major depression (Table 2-2). It is characterized by emotional changes, primarily depressed mood, and by vegetative changes, consisting of alterations in sleep, appetite, and energy levels.

Epidemiology

The lifetime prevalence (will occur at some point in a person's life) rate for major depressive disorder is 5% to

TABLE 2-1

Classification of Mood Disorders

Unipolar	Bipolar	Etiologic
Major depressive disorder	Bipolar I disorder	Substance-induced mood disorder
Dysthymic disorder	Bipolar II disorder	Mood disorder due to general medical condition
	Cyclothymic disorder	

TABLE 2-2

Criteria for Major Depressive Episode

Mood: depressed mood most of the day, nearly every day
Sleep: insomnia or hypersomnia
Interest: marked decrease in interest and pleasure in most activities
Guilt: worthlessness or inappropriate guilt
Energy: fatigue or low energy nearly every day
Concentration: decreased concentration or increased indecisiveness
Appetite: increased or decreased appetite or weight gain or loss
Psychomotor: psychomotor agitation or retardation
Suicidality: recurrent thoughts of death, suicidal ideation, suicidal plan, suicide attempt

General criteria for a major depressive episode require five or more of the following symptoms present for at least 2 weeks; one symptom must be *depressed mood* or *loss of interest or pleasure*. These symptoms must be a change from prior functioning and cannot be due to a medical condition, cannot be substance induced, and cannot be due to bereavement. The symptoms must also cause *distress or impairment*.

Source: Diagnostic and statistical manual of mental disorders. 4th ed. Mood disorders. Washington, DC: American Psychiatric Association, 1994:327.

20%. The female-to-male ratio is 2:1. Race distributions appear equal, and socioeconomic variables do not seem to be a factor. The incidence (rate of new cases) is greatest between the ages of 20 and 40 and decreases over the age of 65.

Etiology

Psychological theories of depression generally view interpersonal losses (actual or perceived losses) as risk factors for developing depression. In fact, available evidence suggests that childhood loss of a parent or loss of a spouse are associated with depression. Classic psychoanalytic theories center on ambivalence toward the lost object (person), although more recent theories focus on the critical importance of the object relationship in maintaining psychic equilibrium and self-regard. The cognitive behavioral model views cognitive distortions as the primary events that foster a negative misperception of the world, which in turn generate negative emotions. The learned helplessness model (based on animal studies) suggests that depression arises when individuals come to believe they can have no control over the stresses and pains that beset them.

Biologic, familial, and genetic data support the idea of a biologic diathesis in the genesis of depression. Genetic studies show that depression is more common in pairs of monozygotic twins than dizygotic. Unipolar depression in a parent leads to an increased incidence in the offspring of both unipolar and bipolar mood disorders.

Neurotransmitter evidence points to abnormalities in amine neurotransmitters as mediators of depressive states: The evidence is strongest for deficiencies in norepinephrine and serotonin.

Neuroendocrine abnormalities in the hypothalamic-pituitary-adrenal axis are often present in depression and suggest a neuroendocrine link.

Sleep disturbances are near universal complaints in depressed persons. Objective evidence from sleep studies reveals that deep sleep (delta sleep, stages 3 and 4) is decreased in depression and that rapid-eye-movement (REM) sleep alterations include increased time spent in REM and earlier onset of REM in the sleep cycle (decreased latency to REM).

Clinical Manifestations

History and Mental Status Examination A major depressive disorder is diagnosed if a patient has at least one episode of major depression and does not meet criteria for bipolar disorder or etiologic mood disorder. Major depression is characterized by emotional and vegetative changes. Emotional changes most commonly include depressed mood with feelings of sadness, hopelessness, guilt, and despair. Irritability of mood may be the primary mood complaint in some cases. Vegetative symptoms include alterations in sleep, appetite, energy, and libido.

Major depression is frequently **recurrent**. The usual duration of an untreated episode (Fig. 2-1A) is 6 to 12 months. **Fifteen percent** of patients diagnosed with major depression die by suicide at some point in their lifetime. (highest x)

Differential Diagnosis Mood disorders secondary to (induced by) medical illnesses or substance abuse are the primary differential diagnoses. Psychotic depression must be differentiated from schizophrenia; negative symptoms of schizophrenia can mimic depression. Persons with major depression may eventually meet criteria for bipolar disorder.

Management

Depression is responsive to **psychotherapy** and **pharmacotherapy**. Milder cases may be treated with brief psychotherapy interventions alone. For more severe cases, antidepressant medications combined with psychotherapy are superior to medications or psychotherapy alone. Among the psychotherapies, supportive, cognitive-behavioral, and brief interpersonal therapies have the most data to support their efficacy. There is a long tradition of psychodynamic psychotherapy in treating depression, which, although not empirically well studied, is an established form of treatment.

There are many classes of antidepressants available that are effective and are usually chosen according to side-effect profiles. Presently, available classes of antidepressants include tricyclic antidepressants, selective serotonin reuptake inhibitors, monoamine oxidase inhibitors, and atypical antidepressants. In addition, lithium, thyroid hormone, and psychostimulants may be used as augmentative treatments. Electroconvulsive therapy (ECT) is used in psychotic, severe, or treatment refractory depressions or when medications are contraindicated (e.g., in the elderly or debilitated). Antipsychotic medications are an essential adjunct to antidepressants in psychotic depressions. Anxiolytics

Figure 2-1 Unipolar mood disorders. (A) Major depressive disorder and (B) dysthymic disorder.

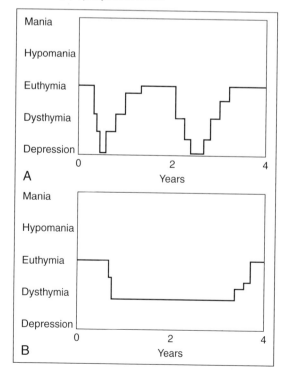

may be used as adjuncts to antidepressants in depression with high levels of anxiety, although more sedating antidepressants may suffice. Phototherapy can be used for seasonal mood disorders.

Key Points
Major depression

1. Is a unipolar mood disorder;
2. Is often recurrent;
3. Has a 15% suicide rate;
4. Is best treated with combined psychotherapy and pharmacotherapy.

Dysthymic Disorder
Dysthymic disorder is a mild chronic form of major depression.

Epidemiology
The lifetime prevalence is 6%.

Etiology
Because dysthymia is often conceptualized as a milder chronic form of major depression, similar etiologies are generally attributed to dysthymia.

Clinical Manifestations
History and Mental Status Examination Dysthymic disorder is a chronic and less severe form of major depression. The diagnosis of dysthymia requires a minimum of 2 years of chronically depressed mood most of the time (Fig. 2-1B). Associated symptoms and complaints may include change in appetite and sleep, fatigue, decreased concentration, and hopelessness. Dysthymia can be chronic and difficult to treat. At times, major depressive episodes may co-occur, giving rise to the term double depression.

Differential Diagnosis Major depression and etiologic mood disorders are the major differential diagnostic considerations.

Management
Treatment is similar to major depression except that psychotherapy may play a larger role and the course of treatment may be more protracted.

Key Points
Dysthymia

1. Is a unipolar mood disorder;
2. Is chronic, lasting at least 2 years;
3. Is often treatment refractory.

▶ BIPOLAR DISORDERS
The bipolar disorders are bipolar I disorder, bipolar II disorder, and cyclothymia.

Bipolar I Disorder
Bipolar I disorder is the most serious of the bipolar disorders and is diagnosed after at least one episode of mania (Table 2-3). Patients with bipolar I disorder typically also have major depressive episodes in the course of their lives.

Epidemiology
The lifetime prevalence is 0.4% to 1.6% and the male-to-female ratio is equal. There are no racial variations in incidence.

Etiology
Genetic and familial studies reveal that bipolar I disorder is associated with increased bipolar I, bipolar II, and major depressive disorders in first-degree relatives. X linkage has been demonstrated in some studies but remains controversial. Mania can be precipitated by psychosocial stressors, and there is evidence that sleep/wake cycle perturbations may predispose to mania.

Clinical Manifestations
History and Mental Status Examination Bipolar I disorder is defined by the occurrence of mania (or a mixed episode). A single manic episode is sufficient

---

TABLE 2-3
Criteria for Manic Episode

Three to four of the following criteria are required during the elevated mood period:

Self-esteem: highly inflated, grandiosity
Sleep: decreased need for sleep, rested after only a few hours
Speech: pressured
Thoughts: racing thoughts and flight of ideas
Attention: easy distractibility
Activity: increased goal directed activity
Hedonism: high excess involvement in pleasurable activities (sex, spending, travel)

General criteria for a manic episode require a clear period of persistently *elevated, expansive, or irritable mood* lasting 1 week or severe enough to require hospitalization. These symptoms must be a change from prior functioning and cannot be due to a medical condition and cannot be substance induced. The symptoms also must cause *distress or impairment*.
Source: Diagnostic and statistical manual of mental disorders. 4th ed. Mood disorders. Washington, DC: American Psychiatric Association, 1994:332.

to meet diagnostic requirements; most patients, however, have **recurrent** episodes of mania typically intermixed with depressive episodes. The criteria for a manic episode are outlined in Table 2-3.

The first episode of mania usually occurs in the early 20s. Manic episodes are typically <u>briefer</u> than depressive episodes. The transition between mania and depression occurs without an intervening period of euthymia in about two of three patients (Fig. 2-2A). Lifetime suicide rates range from 10% to 15%.

Differential Diagnosis Mania may be induced by antidepressant treatment, including antidepressant

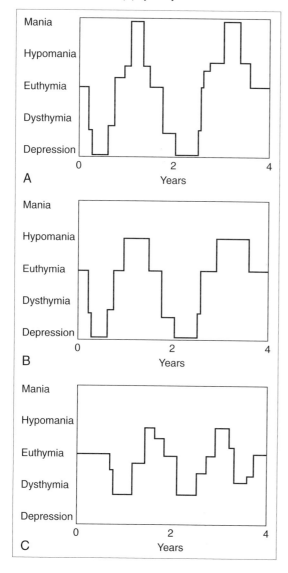

Figure 2-2 Bipolar mood disorders. (A) Bipolar I disorder, (B) bipolar II disorder, and (C) cyclothymia.

medications, psychostimulants, ECT, and phototherapy. When this occurs, the patient is diagnosed with substance-induced mood disorder, not bipolar disorder. Mood disorder due to a general medical condition is the other major differential consideration. Schizoaffective disorder, <u>borderline personality disorder</u>, and <u>depression with agitation</u> are also considerations.

Management

The mainstay of treatment for acute mania is **antipsychotics** in conjunction with **benzodiazepines** (for rapid tranquilization) and **mood stabilizers.** Antipsychotics are frequently used in mania with and without psychotic features. Lithium is the most commonly used mood stabilizer, but valproic acid is quite effective, recently U.S. Food and Drug Administration approved, and is more effective for the rapid cycling variant of mania. Carbamazepine and long-acting benzodiazepines are used if first-line treatments fail. ECT is used in patients with medication intolerance and where a more immediate response is medically or psychiatrically needed.

Mood stabilizer maintenance therapy is essential in preventing the recurrence of mania and also appears to decrease the recurrence of depression. Psychotherapy is used to encourage medication compliance, to help patients come to terms with their illness, and to help repair some of the interpersonal damage done while ill (e.g., infidelity, hostility, squandering money). Care must be taken in prescribing antidepressants for depression or dysthymia because of their role in prompting more severe or more frequent manic episodes.

Key Points
Bipolar I disorder

1. Is a biphasic mood disorder;
2. Is cyclic;
3. Has a suicide rate of 10% to 15%;
4. Requires maintenance treatment with mood stabilizers.

Bipolar II Disorder

Bipolar II disorder is similar to bipolar I disorder with the exception that mania is absent in bipolar II disorder and **hypomania** (a milder form of elevated mood than mania) is the essential diagnostic finding.

Epidemiology

Lifetime prevalence is about 0.5%. Bipolar II disorder may be <u>more common in women.</u>

Etiology

Current evidence implicates the same factors as for bipolar I.

Clinical Manifestations

History and Mental Status Examination Bipolar II disorder is characterized by the occurrence of hypomania and episodes of major depression in an individual who has never met criteria for mania or a mixed state. Hypomania is determined by the same symptom complex as mania but the symptoms are less severe, cause less impairment, and usually do not require hospitalization. Bipolar II disorder is **cyclic** (Fig. 2-2B for course of untreated bipolar II). Suicide occurs in **10% to 15%.**

Differential Diagnosis Same as for bipolar I.

Management

Treatment is the same as for bipolar I disorder, although hypomanic episodes typically do not require as aggressive a treatment regimen as mania. Care must be taken in prescribing antidepressants for depression or dysthymia because of their role in prompting more severe or frequent hypomanic episodes.

Key Points

Bipolar II disorder

1. Is a biphasic mood disorder with hypomania;
2. Is recurrent;
3. Has a suicide rate of 10% to 15%.

Cyclothymic Disorder

Cyclothymia is a recurrent, chronic, mild form of bipolar disorder in which mood typically oscillates between hypomania and dysthymia. It is not diagnosed if a person has had either a manic episode or a major depressive episode.

Epidemiology

The lifetime prevalence of cyclothymia is 0.4% to 1%. The rate appears equal in men and women, though women more often seek treatment.

Etiology

Familial and genetic evidence reveals a familial increase in other mood disorders.

Clinical Manifestations

History and Mental Status Examination Cyclothymia is a milder form of bipolar disorder consisting of **recurrent mood disturbances** between hypomania and dysthymic mood. A single episode of hypomania is sufficient to diagnose cyclothymia; however, most individuals also have dysthymic periods. The diagnosis of cyclothymia is **never** made when there is a history of **mania** or **major depressive episode** or **mixed episode**. The course of untreated cyclothymia is depicted in Figure 2-2C.

Differential Diagnosis The principal differential is among other unipolar and bipolar mood disorders, substance-induced mood disorder, and mood disorder due to a general medical condition. Personality disorders (especially borderline) with labile mood may be confused with cyclothymia.

Management

Psychotherapy, mood stabilizers, and antidepressants are used.

Key Points

Cyclothymia

1. Is a biphasic mood disorder without frank mania or depression; Hypomania + Dysthymia
2. Is chronic and recurrent.

▶ MOOD DISORDERS WITH KNOWN ETIOLOGY

Substance-Induced Mood Disorder

Substance-induced mood disorder is diagnosed when medications, other psychoactive substances, ECT, or phototherapy are proximate events and the likely cause of the mood disturbance. All aforementioned types of mood disorder (i.e., unipolar, bipolar) may occur.

Mood Disorder Due To a General Medical Condition

This category is for mood disturbances apparently caused by a medical illness. Endocrine disorders, such as thyroid and adrenal dysfunction, are common etiologies. Postpartum mood disorders are excluded from this criteria; they are modifiers of unipolar and bipolar mood disorders (see above).

▶ SUBTYPES AND MODIFIERS

Various diagnostic specifiers can be applied to specific subtypes of mood disorders. These have prognostic and treatment implications and may prove to have etiologic implications.

Melancholic: Melancholic depression is a severe form of depression associated with guilt, remorse, loss of pleasure, and extreme vegetative symptoms.

Postpartum: Postpartum depression occurs within 4 weeks of delivery. The presence of one episode of postpartum mood disorder is strongly predictive of a recurrence.

Seasonal: Seasonal mood disorders show a consistent seasonal pattern of variation. The most common pattern is a worsening of depression during the fall and winter with improvement in the spring. The reverse is sometimes true. If the depression is a component of a bipolar disorder, the manic and hypomanic episodes may show a seasonal association.

Atypical: Atypical depressions show a pattern of hypersomnia, increased appetite or weight gain, mood reactivity, long-standing rejection sensitivity, anergia, and leaden paralysis.

Rapid Cycling: Patients with bipolar disorder may have frequent (rapid) cycles. To meet criteria for rapid cycling, four mood disturbances per year must be present. The suicide rate may be higher than in non-rapid cyclers. *give Depakoate*

Catatonic: The catatonic specifier is applied to mood disorders when there are pronounced movement abnormalities, including motoric immobility or excessive purposeless motor activity, maintenance of a rigid posture, mutism, stereotyped movement, echolalia (repetition of a word or phrase just spoken by another person), or echopraxia (repetition of movements made by another person).

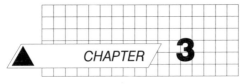

CHAPTER 3

Anxiety Disorders

The term **anxiety** refers to many different entities in which the sufferer experiences a sense of impending threat or doom that is not well defined or realistically based. Anxiety can be adaptive or pathologic, transient or chronic, and is manifested in a variety of psychological and physical states. **Anxiety disorders** are a heterogeneous group of disorders in which the feeling of anxiety is the major element. They are the most prevalent group of psychiatric disorders; according to the Epidemiological Catchment Area study, 7.3% of all Americans meet *The Diagnostic and Statistical Manual of Mental Disorders*, 3rd edition (DSM-III; the DSM version used at the time) criteria at a given point in time (so-called point prevalence). Anxiety disorders listed in the DSM-IV are shown in Table 3-1.

▶ PANIC DISORDER AND AGORAPHOBIA

Panic disorder is characterized by recurrent unexpected panic attacks that can occur *with or without* agoraphobia. Agoraphobia is a disabling condition in which patients fear places in which escape might be difficult. Whether occurring as distinct entities or together, panic disorder and agoraphobia are common, sometimes disabling, conditions.

Epidemiology Women > men.

Panic disorder occurs more frequently in women, with a lifetime prevalence of 2% to 3%. The typical onset is in the 20s, with most cases beginning before age 30.

Agoraphobia also occurs more frequently in women, with a lifetime prevalence of between 2% and 6%. Only one-third of patients with agoraphobia also have panic disorder. However, most patients with agoraphobia seen clinically also have panic disorder. This apparent contradiction is due to the fact that patients with agoraphobia alone are unlikely to seek treatment.

Etiology

The etiology of panic disorder is unknown. There are several popular biologic theories involving CO_2 hypersensitivity, abnormalities in lactate metabolism, an abnormality of the locus coeruleus (a region in the brain that regulates level of arousal), and elevated central nervous system catecholamine levels. The gamma-amino butyric acid (GABA) receptor also has been implicated as etiologic because of the response of patients to benzodiazepines and the ability to induce panic with GABA antagonists in patients with anxiety disorders.

Learning theorists posit that panic attacks are a conditioned response to a fearful situation. For example, a person has an automobile accident and experiences severe anxiety, including palpitations. Thereafter, palpitations alone, experienced during exercise or any sympathetic nervous system response, may induce the conditioned response of a panic attack.

Clinical Manifestations

History and Mental Status Examination

Panic disorder is characterized by **recurrent unexpected panic attacks** that can occur **with or without** agoraphobia (see below). Panic attacks typically come on suddenly, peak within minutes, and last 5 to 30 minutes. The patient must experience 4 of 13 typical symptoms of panic outlined in Table 3-2.

To warrant the diagnosis, one of the following must occur for at least 1 month: persistent concern about having additional attacks, worry about the implications of the attack (losing control, "going crazy"), or a significant change of behavior related to the attacks (e.g., restriction of activities).

Agoraphobia is a disabling complication of panic disorder but also can occur in patients with no history of panic disorder. It is characterized by an **intense fear of places or situations** in which escape might be difficult (or embarrassing). Patients with agoraphobia and panic disorder typically fear having a panic attack in a public place and being embarrassed or unable to escape. Those with agoraphobia alone (two-thirds of those with agoraphobia) simply avoid public arenas but do not have panic attacks. Although some agoraphobic patients are so disabled that they are homebound, many are comforted by the presence of a companion, allowing them to enter some public places with less anxiety.

Differential Diagnosis

Panic attacks should be distinguished from the direct physiologic effects of a substance or a general medical

TABLE 3-1

Anxiety Disorders

Panic disorder *with* agoraphobia	Generalized anxiety disorder
Panic disorder *without* agoraphobia	Acute stress disorder
Agoraphobia	Posttraumatic stress disorder
Social phobia	Substance-induced anxiety disorder
Specific phobia	Anxiety disorder due to a general medical condition
Obsessive-compulsive disorder	Anxiety disorder not otherwise specified

TABLE 3-2

DSM-IV Criteria for Panic Attack

A discrete period of intense fear or discomfort, in which <u>four</u> (or more) of the following symptoms developed abruptly and reached a <u>peak within 10 minutes:</u>

▲ Palpitations, pounding heart, or accelerated heart rate
▲ Sweating
▲ Trembling or shaking
▲ Sensations of shortness of breath or smothering
▲ Feeling of choking
▲ Chest pain or discomfort
▲ Nausea or abdominal distress
▲ Feeling dizzy, unsteady, lightheaded, or faint
▲ Derealization (feelings of unreality) or depersonalization (being detached from oneself)
▲ Fear of losing control or going crazy
▲ Fear of dying
▲ *Numbing sensation of hands or Extremities*

Adapted from *Diagnostic and Statistical Manual of Mental Disorders,* 4th edition. Anxiety disorders. Washington, DC: American Psychiatric Association, 1994:395.

condition. The panic attacks also cannot be accounted for by another mental disorder (such as social phobia or obsessive-compulsive disorder).

Management

Not surprisingly, the main treatments of panic disorder are pharmacotherapy and cognitive-behavioral therapy or their combination. Specific **tricyclic antidepressants** (TCAs), specific **monoamine oxidase inhibitors** (MAOIs), **selective serotonin reuptake inhibitors** (SSRIs), and high-potency **benzodiazepines** have been shown to be effective in controlled studies. **Cognitive-behavioral therapy** involves the use of relaxation exercises and <u>desensitization</u> combined with education aimed at helping the patient to understand that their panic attacks are a result of misinterpretation of bodily sensations. The patient can thereby learn that the sensations are innocuous and self-limited, which diminishes the panicky response. **Exposure therapy,** in which the patient <u>incrementally</u> confronts

a feared stimulus, has been shown to be effective in treating agoraphobia.

Key Points

Panic disorder

1. Is characterized by recurrent <u>unexpected</u> panic attacks;
2. Can be seen with or without agoraphobia;
3. Is treated with antidepressants and benzodiazepines with cognitive-behavioral techniques. *(CBT)*

Agoraphobia

1. Is fear of not being able to (or being too embarrassed to) escape a place or situation;
2. Can be a complication of panic disorder;
3. Most often occurs alone (without panic);
4. Is treated with exposure therapy. *D.O.C = SSRI*
   PRN = BDZ / Buspar.

▶ SPECIFIC PHOBIA

Specific phobia is an anxiety disorder characterized by intense fear of particular objects or situations (e.g., snakes, heights). <u>It is the most common psychiatric disorder.</u>

Epidemiology   *Women > men.*

Specific phobias are more prevalent <u>in women</u> than men and occur with a lifetime prevalence of 25%. Typical onset is in childhood, with most cases occurring <u>before age 12.</u>

Etiology

Phobic disorders, including specific phobia, tend to run in families. Behavioral theorists argue that phobias are learned by being paired with traumatic events.

Clinical Manifestations

History and Mental Status Examination

A phobia is an irrational fear of a specific object, place, activity, or situation that is out of proportion to any actual danger. To meet the DSM-IV criteria for specific phobia, a patient must experience a marked persistent fear that is recognized by the patient to be excessive or unreasonable and is cued by the presence or anticipation of a specific object or situation; exposure to the stimulus must almost invariably provoke the anxiety reaction; and the avoidance or distress over the feared situation must impair everyday activities or relationships. For those <u>under age 18,</u> symptoms must persist for at <u>least 6 months.</u>

Differential Diagnosis

The principal differential diagnosis is another mental disorder (such as avoidance of school in separation anxiety disorder) presenting with anxiety or fearfulness.

Management

Specific childhood phobias tend to remit spontaneously with age. When they persist into adulthood, they often become chronic. However, they rarely cause disability. Exposure therapy in the form of **systematic desensitization** or **flooding** is the treatment of choice. There is no role for medication.

Key Points

Specific phobia

1. Is an intense fear of a certain object, place, activity, or situation;

2. Occurs in 25% of the population at some point in their lifetime;

3. Usually has an onset before age 12;

4. Is treated with systematic desensitization and flooding.

► SOCIAL PHOBIA

Social phobia is an anxiety disorder in which patients have an intense fear of being scrutinized in social or public situations (e.g., giving a speech, speaking in class). The disorder may be **generalized** or **limited** to specific situations.

Epidemiology

Social phobias occur equally among men and women and affect 3% to 5% of the population. The typical onset is in adolescence, with most cases occurring before age 25.

Etiology

Phobic disorders, including social phobia, tend to run in families. Behavioral theorists argue that phobias are learned by being paired with traumatic events. Some theorists posit that hypersensitivity to rejection is a psychological antecedent of social phobia.

Clinical Manifestations

History and Mental Status Examination

Social phobias are characterized by the fear of situations in which the person is exposed to **unfamiliar people** or to **possible scrutiny** by others. Exposure to the feared social situation must almost invariably provoke an anxiety reaction. Avoidance or distress over the feared situation must impair everyday activities or relationships. For those under age 18, symptoms must persist for at least 6 months. It can either be generalized (the patient fears nearly all situations) or limited to specific situations.

Differential Diagnosis

The principal differential diagnosis is another mental disorder (such as avoidance of school in separation anxiety disorder) presenting with anxiety or fearfulness.

Management

Mild cases of social phobia can be treated with **cognitive-behavioral therapy**, but many cases require **medication**. Monoamine oxidase inhibitors, beta-blockers, selective serotonin reuptake inhibitors, and alprazolam have been shown to treat social phobia. Cognitive-behavioral therapy uses the exposure therapy techniques of flooding and systematic desensitization to reduce anxiety in feared situations. Supportive individual and group psychotherapy is helpful to restore self-esteem and to encourage venturing into feared situations.

Key Points

Social phobia

1. Is fear of exposure to scrutiny by others;

2. Has a lifetime prevalence of 3% to 5%;

3. Typically occurs before age 25;

4. Can be generalized or limited;

5. Is treated with MAOIs, SSRIs, beta-blockers, or benzodiazepines and with cognitive-behavioral therapy.

► GENERALIZED ANXIETY DISORDER

Generalized anxiety disorder (GAD) is characterized by intense pervasive worry over virtually every aspect of life associated with **physical manifestations** of anxiety.

Epidemiology

The lifetime prevalence of generalized anxiety disorder is approximately 5%. The typical age of onset is in the early 20s, but the disorder may begin at any age.

Etiology

Twin studies suggest that GAD has both inherited and environmental etiologies. Serotonergic, noradrenergic, and GABAergic neurotransmitter systems have been studied in relation to GAD, but the biologic etiology remains obscure. Learning theorists posit that GAD is due to cognitive distortions in which patients misperceive situations as dangerous when they are not.

Clinical Manifestations

History and Mental Status Examination

Patients with generalized anxiety disorder worry excessively about virtually every aspect of their life (job performance, health, marital relations, and social life). They do not have panic attacks, phobias, obsessions, or compulsions, rather they experience pervasive anxiety and worry (apprehensive expectation) about a number of events or activities that occur most days for at least 6 months. They must also have difficulty **controlling** the worry, and it must be associated with at least three of the following symptoms: restlessness, easily fatigued, difficulty concentrating or mind going blank, irritability, muscle tension, and sleep disturbance.

Differential Diagnosis

The focus of the anxiety and worry in GAD must not be symptomatic of another axis I disorder. For example, the anxiety and worry cannot be about having a panic attack (as in panic disorder) or being embarrassed in public (as in social phobia).

Management

The pharmacologic treatment of GAD is with **benzodiazepines**, **buspirone** (a nonbenzodiazepine anxiolytic), or **beta-blockers**. Although benzodiazepines are very effective, the duration of treatment is limited by the risk of tolerance and dependence. **Relaxation** techniques are also used in the treatment with some success.

Key Points

Generalized anxiety disorder *at least 6 months.*

1. Is intense worry over every aspect of life;
2. Is characterized by difficulty controlling the worry;
3. Is associated with physical manifestations of anxiety;
4. Is treated with benzodiazepine, buspirone, beta-blockers, and relaxation techniques.

▶ POSTTRAUMATIC STRESS DISORDER

Posttraumatic stress disorder (PTSD) is an anxiety disorder characterized by the persistent re-experience of a trauma, efforts to avoid recollecting the trauma, and hyperarousal.

TABLE 3-3

Posttraumatic Stress Disorder

Re-experience of the trauma.
Efforts to avoid recollection of the trauma.
Hyperarousal.

Epidemiology

The prevalence of PTSD is estimated at 0.5% among men and 1.2% among women. The typical male experience is through combat; the typical female experience is through violence or rape. PTSD may occur at any age from childhood through adulthood and may begin hours, days, or even years after the initial trauma.

Etiology

The central etiologic factor in PTSD is the trauma. There may be some necessary predisposition to PTSD because all people who experience similar traumas do not develop the syndrome.

Clinical Manifestations

History and Mental Status Examination

People with PTSD have endured a **traumatic event** (e.g., combat, physical assault, rape, explosion) in which the person experienced, witnessed, or was confronted with actual or potential death, serious physical injury, or a threat to physical integrity. The traumatic event is subsequently re-experienced through repetitive intrusive images or dreams or through recurrent illusions, hallucinations, or flashbacks of the event. In an adaptive attempt, these patients make efforts to **avoid recollections** of the event often through psychological mechanisms (e.g., dissociation, numbing) or actual avoidance of circumstances that will evoke recall. They also experience feelings of detachment from others and exhibit evidence of autonomic hyperarousal (e.g., difficulty sleeping, exaggerated startle response).

Differential Diagnosis

Symptoms that resemble PTSD may be seen in depression, generalized anxiety disorder, panic disorder, obsessive compulsive disorder, and dissociative disorder. When symptoms resemble PTSD, ensure that there also are symptoms from all three categories of symptoms; if not, consider one of the above diagnoses.

Management

Treatment is with a combination of symptom-directed psychopharmacologic agents and psychotherapy (individual or group). TCAs and MAOIs are the most commonly used medications in PTSD, especially when there is a comorbid major depression. SSRIs have also been used. **Psychotherapy** is typically tailored to the nature of the trauma, degree of coping skills, and the support systems available to the patient.

Key Points

Posttraumatic stress disorder

1. Is a response to trauma;
2. Is characterized by re-experience of the trauma, efforts to avoid recalling the trauma, and hyper-arousal;
3. Is treated with medications directed at specific symptoms and with psychotherapy. *TCA/MAOI*

▶ OBSESSIVE-COMPULSIVE DISORDER

Obsessive-compulsive disorder (OCD) is an anxiety disorder in which patients experience recurrent obsessions and compulsions that cause significant distress and occupy a significant portion of the affected person's life.

Epidemiology

The lifetime prevalence of OCD is 2% to 3%. Typical onset of the disorder is between the late teens and early 20s, but one-third of patients show symptoms of OCD before age 15.

Etiology *5-HT, Conditioning*

Behavioral models of OCD claim that obsessions and compulsions are produced and sustained through classic and operant conditioning. Interestingly, OCD is seen more frequently after brain injury or disease (e.g., head trauma, seizure disorders, Huntington's disease), and twin studies show that monozygotic twins have a higher concordance rate than dizygotic twins; these findings support a biologic basis for the disorder. The neurotransmitter serotonin has been implicated as a mediator in obsessive thinking and compulsive behaviors.

Clinical Manifestations

History and Mental Status Examination

Patients with OCD experience obsessions and compulsions. **Obsessions** are recurrent intrusive ideas, thoughts, or images that cause significant anxiety and distress; **compulsions** are repetitive purposeful physical or mental actions that generally are performed in response to obsessions. The compulsive "rituals" are meant to neutralize the obsessions, diminish anxiety, or somehow magically prevent a dreaded event or situation.

Differential Diagnosis

It is important to distinguish the **obsessional** thinking of OCD from the **delusional** thinking of schizophrenia or other psychotic disorders. Obsessions are usually unwanted, resisted, and recognized by the patient as coming from their own thoughts, whereas delusions are generally regarded by the patient to be distinct from his or her thoughts and typically are not resisted. For example, patients with depression often experience obsessive ruminations that can be distinguished from obsessions because they are transient and not considered unwanted nor are they resisted.

Management

Clomipramine, fluvoxamine, and **SSRIs** have been shown to be quite effective in treating OCD. Although poorly studied, the behavioral techniques of **systematic desensitization** and **flooding** and response prevention have been used successfully to treat compulsive rituals. For example, someone who fears contamination from an object will hold the object repeatedly in therapy while simultaneously being prevented from carrying out the ritual associated with the dreaded object.

Key Points

Obsessive-compulsive disorder

1. Is characterized by recurrent obsessions and compulsions;
2. Causes distress and wastes time by carrying out the obsessions/compulsions/rituals;
3. Has a lifetime prevalence of 2% to 3%;
4. Is treated with clomipramine, fluvoxamine, and SSRIs and with systematic desensitization and flooding.

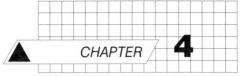

CHAPTER 4

AxisII # Personality Disorders

𝒫ersonality disorders are coded on Axis II in the *Diagnostic and Statistical Manual of Mental Disorders*, 4th edition (DSM-IV). Ten different types of personality disorders are grouped into clusters based on similar overall characteristics. There are **three** recognized personality disorder clusters: **odd and eccentric, dramatic and emotional**, and **anxious and fearful** (Table 4-1).

DSM-IV general diagnostic criteria for personality disorders are outlined in Table 4-2. Criteria for individual personality disorders are discussed below. Personality disorders frequently overlap in symptoms.

▶ CLUSTER A (ODD AND ECCENTRIC)

Paranoid Personality Disorder
People with paranoid personality disorder are distrustful and suspicious and anticipate harm and betrayal.

Epidemiology
Paranoid personality disorder has a lifetime prevalence of 0.5% to 2.5% of the general population. Relatives of chronic schizophrenics and patients with persecutory delusional disorders show an increased prevalence of paranoid personality disorder.

Etiology
Environmental precursors are unclear. Family studies suggest a link to delusional disorder (paranoid type). There appears to be a small increase in relatives of schizophrenics.

Clinical Manifestations
History and Mental Status Examination People with paranoid personality disorder are distrustful and suspicious and see the world as malevolent. They anticipate harm, betrayal, and deception. Not surprisingly, they are not forthcoming about themselves. Give them the emotional distance they psychologically require.

Differential Diagnosis The key distinction is to separate paranoia associated with psychotic disorders from paranoid personality disorder, especially because paranoia associated with psychotic disorders is generally responsive to antipsychotic medications.

Schizoid Personality Disorder
Individuals with schizoid personality disorder are emotionally detached and prefer to be left alone.

Epidemiology
Estimates of lifetime prevalence range as high as 7.5% of the general population, but because they are avoidant of others, they are not commonly seen in clinical practice.

Etiology
There is some evidence to suggest increased prevalence of schizoid personality disorder in relatives of persons with schizophrenia or schizotypal personality disorder. Unloving or neglectful parenting is hypothesized to play a role.

Clinical Manifestations
History and Mental Status Examination These people are loners. They are aloof and detached and have profound difficulty experiencing or expressing emotion. Although they prefer to be left alone and generally do not seek relationships, they may maintain an important bond with a family member.

Differential Diagnosis Schizoid personality disorder can be distinguished from avoidant personality disorder (see below) and social phobia by the fact that schizoid individuals do not seek relationships. Avoidant and socially phobic persons desire relationships, but their anxiety handicaps their capacity to achieve relatedness. Schizophrenia, autistic disorder, and Asperger's disease (a less severe variant of autism) "Gout" clerk: are also differential diagnostic conditions.

Schizotypal Personality Disorder
Individuals with schizotypal personality disorder have odd thought, affect, perception, and beliefs.

Epidemiology
Lifetime prevalence is 3% of the general population.

Etiology
Studies demonstrate intrafamilial aggregation of this disorder, especially among first-degree relatives of schizophrenics.

TABLE 4-1

Classification of Personality Disorders

Cluster A (Odd/Eccentric)	Cluster B (Dramatic/ Emotional)	Cluster C (Anxious/Fearful)
Paranoid	Antisocial	Avoidant
Schizoid	Borderline	Dependent
Schizotypal	Histrionic	Obsessive compulsive
	Narcissistic	

TABLE 4-1

General Diagnostic Criteria for Personality Disorders

Personality disorder patients evidence an enduring pattern of inner experience and behavior, established by adolescence or early adulthood, that:
1. Deviates markedly from cultural expectations
2. Is inflexible and personally and socially pervasive
3. Causes distress or social or work impairment
4. Is a stable pattern of experience and behavior of long duration ("stably unstable")
5. Cannot be explained by another mental illness
6. Is not caused by substance use or medical condition

NOTE: Individuals with personality disorders usually maintain intact reality testing. However, they may have transient psychotic symptoms when stressed by real (or imagined) loss or frustration. Personality disorders are different from personality traits which are typically adaptive, culturally acceptable, and do not cause significant distress or impairment.
Source: From Diagnostic and statistical manual of mental disorders, 4th ed. Mood disorders. Washington, DC: American Psychiatric Association, 1994:633.

Clinical Manifestations

History and Mental Status Examination Schizotypal personality disorder is best thought of as similar to schizophrenia but less severe and without sustained psychotic symptoms. People with this disorder have few relationships and demonstrate oddities of thought, affect, perception, and belief. Many are highly distrustful and often paranoid, which results in a very constricted social world. The lifetime suicide rate among this population is 10%.

Differential Diagnosis Schizophrenia, delusional disorder, and mood disorder with psychosis are the major differential diagnoses.

► CLUSTER B (DRAMATIC AND EMOTIONAL)

Antisocial Personality Disorder

Individuals with antisocial personality (ASP) disorder repetitively disregard the rules and laws of society and rarely experience remorse for their actions.

Epidemiology _Men > Women._

Antisocial personality disorder is present in 3% of men and 1% of women. About half have been arrested; about half of those in prison have ASP.

Etiology

ASP is more common among first-degree relatives of those diagnosed with ASP. In families of an individual with ASP, men show higher rates of ASP and substance abuse, whereas women have higher rates of somatization disorder. A harsh, violent, and criminal environmental so predisposes to this disorder.

Clinical Manifestations

History and Mental Status Examination Individuals with ASP disorder display a flagrant or well-concealed disregard for the rules and laws of society. They are exploitative, lie frequently, endanger others, are impulsive and aggressive, and rarely experience remorse for the harm they cause others. Alcoholism is a frequently associated finding in this population. Many individuals with ASP are indicted or jailed for their actions. Their lifetime suicide risk is 5%.

Differential Diagnosis Bipolar disorder and substance abuse disorder can prompt antisocial behaviors during the acute illness that remit when the disorder is controlled. The antisocial behavior of individuals with ASP, conversely, is not state dependent.

Borderline Personality Disorder

Individuals with borderline personality disorder suffer from instability in relationships, self-image, affect, and impulse control.

Epidemiology

Lifetime prevalence is 1% to 2% of the general population.

Etiology

Borderline personality disorder is about five times as common among first-degree relatives of borderline patients. In addition, this disorder shows increased rates in families of alcoholics and families of individuals with antisocial personality disorder, as well as in families with mood disorders. Females with borderline personality disorder frequently have suffered from sexual or physical abuse or both.

Clinical Manifestations

History and Mental Status Examination Individuals with borderline personality disorder suffer from a legion of symptoms. Their relationships are infused with anger, fear of abandonment, and shifting idealization and devaluation. Their self-image is inchoate, fragmented, and unstable with consequent unpredictable changes in relationships, goals, and values. They are affectively unstable and reactive, with anger, depression, and panic prominent. Their impulsiveness can result in many unsafe behaviors, including drug use, promiscuity, gambling, and other risk-taking behavior. Their self-destructive urges result in frequent suicidal and parasuicidal behavior (behaviors such as superficial cutting or burning or nonfatal overdoses in which the intent is not lethal). They also demonstrate brief paranoia and dissociative symptoms. Suicide attempts can be frequent before the age of 30, and suicide rates approach 10% over a lifetime. The principal intrapsychic defenses they use are primitive with gross denial, distortion, projection, and splitting prominent. The patients may have a broad range of comorbid illnesses, including substance abuse, mood disorders, and eating disorders.

Differential Diagnosis Mood disorders and behavioral changes due to active substance abuse are the principal differential diagnostic considerations. The diagnostic clues are unstable relationships, unstable self-image, unstable affect, and unstable or impulsive behaviors.

Histrionic Personality Disorder

Individuals with histrionic personality disorder have excessive superficial emotionality and a powerful need for attention.

Epidemiology

Lifetime prevalence is 2% to 3% of the general population. In clinical settings, the diagnosis is most frequently applied to women but may equally affect men and women in the general population.

Etiology

There appears to be a familial link to somatization disorder and to ASP disorder.

Clinical Manifestations

History and Mental Status Examination Individuals with histrionic personality disorder are characterized by their excessive and superficial emotionality and their profound need to be the center of attention at all times. Theatrical behavior dominates with lively and dramatic clothing, exaggerated emotional responses to seemingly insignificant events, and inappropriate flirtatious and seductive behavior across a wide variety of circumstances. Despite their apparent plethora of emotion, these individuals often have difficulty with intimacy, frequently believing their relationships are more intimate than they actually are.

Differential Diagnosis Somatization disorder is the principal differential diagnostic consideration.

Narcissistic Personality Disorder

Individuals with narcissistic personality disorder appear arrogant and entitled but suffer from extremely low self-esteem.

Epidemiology *men > women.*

Lifetime prevalence is estimated at 1% in the general population and 2% to 16% in clinical populations. Fifty percent to 75% of those with this diagnosis are men.

Etiology

The etiology of this disorder is unknown.

Clinical Manifestations

History and Mental Status Examination People with narcissistic personality disorder demonstrate an apparently paradoxical combination of self-centeredness and worthlessness. Their sense of self-importance generally is extravagant, and they demand attention and admiration. Concern or empathy for others is typically absent. They often appear arrogant, exploitative, and entitled. However, despite their inflated sense of self, below their brittle facade lies low self-esteem and intense envy of those whom they regard as more desirable, worthy, or able.

Differential Diagnosis The grandiosity of narcissism can be differentiated from the grandiosity of bipolar disorder by the presence of characteristic mood symptoms in bipolar disorder.

► CLUSTER C (ANXIOUS AND FEARFUL)

Avoidant Personality Disorder

Individuals with avoidant personality disorder desire relationships but avoid them because of the anxiety produced by their sense of inadequacy.

Epidemiology

Lifetime prevalence is 0.5% to 1% of the general population and appears to be of equal prevalence in men and women.

Etiology

There are no conclusive data. The pattern of avoidance may start in infancy.

Clinical Manifestations

History and Mental Status Examination People with avoidant personality disorder experience intense feelings of inadequacy. They are painfully sensitive to criticism, so much so that they are compelled to avoid spending time with people. Their fears of rejection and humiliation are so powerful that to engage in a relationship they seek strong guarantees of acceptance. The essence of this disorder is inadequacy, hypersensitivity to criticism, and consequent social inhibition.

Differential Diagnosis The major diagnostic distinction is between avoidant personality disorder and social phobia, generalized type. + Schizoid .

Dependent Personality Disorder

Individuals with dependent personality disorder are extremely needy of others for emotional support and decision-making.

Epidemiology

Lifetime prevalence is 15% to 20%, 2% to 3% clinically.

Etiology

The etiology is unknown.

Clinical Manifestations

History and Mental Status Examination These people yearn to be cared for. Because of their extreme dependence on others for emotional support and decision-making, they live in great and continuous fear of separation from someone they depend on, hence their submissive and clinging behaviors.

Differential Diagnosis People with dependent personality disorder are similar to individuals with borderline personality disorder in their desire to avoid abandonment but do not exhibit the impulsive behaviors and unstable affect and self-image of the borderline patient.

Obsessive-Compulsive Personality Disorder

These individuals are perfectionists who require a great deal of order and control.

Epidemiology   men > women

The estimated prevalence is 1% in the community. Men are diagnosed with obsessive-compulsive personality disorder twice as frequently as women.

Etiology

The etiology is unknown, but there may be an association with mood and anxiety disorders.

Clinical Manifestations

History and Mental Status Examination Individuals with obsessive-compulsive personality disorder are perfectionists. They require order and control in every dimension of their lives. Their attention to minutiae frequently impairs their ability to finish what they start or to maintain sight of their goals. They are cold and rigid in relationships and make frequent moral judgments; devotion to work often replaces intimacy. They are serious and plodding; even recreation becomes a sober task.

Differential Diagnosis Obsessive-compulsive personality disorder can be differentiated from obsessive-compulsive disorder based on symptom severity.

▶ MANAGEMENT

Because personality may have temperamental components and is developed over a lifetime of interacting with one's environment, **personality disorders** are generally **resistant to treatment.** In general, **psychotherapy** is recommended for most personality disorders. Psychodynamically based therapies are commonly used, although they must be modified to each individual and each disorder. Cognitive, behavioral, and family therapies are also used to treat these disorders. Empirical studies validating the efficacy of various therapies are generally lacking. Dialectical behavioral therapy was developed specifically for the treatment of borderline personality disorder and has been validated in empirical studies. Group therapy incorporating various psychotherapeutic modalities also is used.

Pharmacotherapy is widely used in personality disorders, although no specific medication has been shown to treat any specific disorder. Instead, medications are targeted at the various associated symptoms of personality disorders. For example, mood stabilizers may be used for mood instability and impulsiveness. Benzodiazepines are commonly used for anxiety, although the potential for their abuse and dependence is too often overlooked. Beta blockers are also used frequently. For depression, obsessive-compulsive symptoms and eating disturbances, selective serotonin reuptake inhibitors and other antidepressants have been successfully used. Psychotic or paranoid symptoms are commonly treated with low-dose antipsychotics.

▶ KEY CONCEPTS

Personality disorders

1. Are categorized into three symptom clusters;

2. Are an enduring pattern of experience and behavior;

3. Can produce transient psychotic symptoms during stress;

4. Are treated with psychotherapy and medications targeted at symptom relief;

5. Are treatment refractory;

6. May have genetic associations with Axis I disorders.

OCPD = SSRI - PROZAC, Clomipiramine (Perfectionist - no treatment, exc. psychotherapy)

BORDER = Li/VPA, BDZ for impulsivity.

SCHIZOID or SCHIZOTYPAL = LOW ANTIPSYCH.

CHAPTER 5

Substance-Related Disorders

Substance abuse is as common as it is costly to society. It is etiologic for many medical illnesses and frequently is comorbid with psychiatric illness. The *Diagnostic and Statistical Manual of Mental Disorders,* 4th edition (DSM-IV) defines substance abuse and dependence independent of the substance. Hence, alcohol abuse and dependence is defined by the same criteria as heroin abuse and dependence. This chapter defines abuse and dependence and provides clinical descriptions of each substance-related disorder.

▶ SUBSTANCE ABUSE

The DSM-IV defines substance abuse as a maladaptive pattern of substance use leading to clinically significant impairment or distress as manifested by

▲ Failure to fulfill major role obligations at home, school, or work;

▲ Recurrent substance use in situations in which it is physically hazardous;

▲ Recurrent substance-related legal problems;

▲ Recurrent substance use despite persistent or recurrent social or interpersonal problems caused or exacerbated by the effects of the substance.

The DSM-IV recognizes the different signs and symptoms associated with various drug addictions. We review the common substance-related disorders in sequence.

▶ SUBSTANCE DEPENDENCE

Substance dependence is defined as a maladaptive pattern of substance use leading to clinically significant impairment or distress, as manifested by three (or more) of the following:

1. Tolerance;
2. Withdrawal;
3. Repeated, unintended, excessiveuse;
4. Persistent failed efforts to cut down;
5. Excessive time is spent trying to obtain the substance;
6. Reduction in important social, occupational, or recreational activities;

7. Continued use despite awareness that substance is cause of psychological or physical difficulties.

Although each substance dependence disorder has unique features, these are considered the common features that define substance dependence. Each substance use disorder is discussed, with particular attention to unique features of each disorder.

▶ ALCOHOL-RELATED DISORDERS

Alcohol Intoxication

Alcohol intoxication is defined by the presence of slurred speech, incoordination, unsteady gait, nystagmus, impairment in attention or memory, stupor or coma, and clinically significant maladaptive behavioral or psychological changes (inappropriate sexual or aggressive behavior, mood lability, impaired judgment, impaired social or occupational functioning) that develops during or shortly after alcohol ingestion.

The diagnosis of alcohol intoxication must be differentiated from other medical or neurologic states that may mimic intoxication, for example, diabetic hypoglycemia; toxicity with various agents, including, but not limited to, ethylene glycol, lithium, and phenytoin; and intoxication with benzodiazepines or barbiturates. The diagnosis of alcohol intoxication can be confirmed by serum toxicologic screening, including a blood alcohol level (BAL).

Alcohol Dependence

Alcohol abuse becomes alcohol dependence when **tolerance** and **withdrawal** symptoms develop. The alcohol dependent patient drinks larger amounts over longer periods of time than intended, spends a great deal of time attempting to obtain alcohol, and reduces participation in or eliminates important social, occupational, or recreational activities because of alcohol. In alcohol dependence, there also is a persistent desire or unsuccessful efforts to cut down or control alcohol intake.

Epidemiology

The percentage of Americans who abuse alcohol is thought to be high. Two-thirds of Americans drink occasionally; 12% are heavy drinkers, drinking almost every day and becoming intoxicated several times a month. The Epidemiological Catchment Area study found a lifetime prevalence of alcohol dependence of 14%. The male-to-female prevalence ratio for alcohol dependence is 4:1.

Etiology

The etiology of alcohol dependence is unknown. Adoption studies and monozygotic twin studies demonstrate a partial genetic basis, particularly for men with alcoholism. Male alcoholics are more likely than female alcoholics to have a family history of alcoholism. Compared with control subjects, the relatives of alcoholics are more likely to have higher rates of depression and antisocial personality disorder. Adoption studies also reveal that alcoholism is multidetermined: genetics and environment (family rearing) both play a role.

Clinical Manifestations

History, Physical and Mental Status Examinations, and Laboratory Tests

The alcohol-dependent patient may **deny** and/or **minimize** the extent of drinking, making the early diagnosis of alcoholism difficult. The patient may present with accidents or falls, blackouts, motor vehicle accidents, or after an arrest for driving under the influence. Because denial is so prominent in the disorder, collateral information from family members is essential to the diagnosis. Early physical findings that suggest alcoholism include acne rosacea, palmar erythema, and painless hepatomegaly (from fatty infiltration).

Signs of more advanced alcoholism include cirrhosis, jaundice, ascites, testicular atrophy, gynecomastia, and Dupuytren's contracture. Cirrhosis can lead to complications including variceal bleeding, hepatocellular carcinoma, and hepatic encephalopathy. Medical disorders with an increased incidence in alcohol-dependent patients include pneumonia, tuberculosis, cardiomyopathy, hypertension, and gastrointestinal cancers (i.e., oral, esophageal, rectal, colon, pancreas, and liver).

There also are numerous neuropsychiatric complications of alcoholism. **Wernicke-Korsakoff syndrome** may develop in the alcohol-dependent patient because of **thiamine deficiency.** The Wernicke stage of the syndrome consists of the triad of **nystagmus, ataxia**, and **mental confusion.** These symptoms remit with the injection of thiamine (100 mg IM). Without thiamine, Wernicke encephalopathy may progress to Korsakoff's psychosis (**anterograde amnesia** and **confabulation**),

which is irreversible in two-thirds of patients. Other neuropsychiatric complications of alcoholism include alcoholic hallucinosis, alcohol-induced dementia, peripheral neuropathy, substance-induced depression, and suicide. In the later stages of alcoholism, significant social and occupational impairment is likely: job loss and family estrangement are typical.

Various laboratory tests are also helpful in making the diagnosis. BALs quantitatively confirm alcohol in the serum. They also can provide a rough measure of tolerance. In general, the higher the BAL without significant signs of intoxication, the more tolerant the patient has become of the intoxicating effects of alcohol. Alcohol-dependent patients also develop elevated high-density-lipoprotein cholesterol and decreased low-density-lipoprotein cholesterol, elevated mean corpuscular volume, elevated serum glutamic-oxaloacetic transaminase, and elevated serum glutamic-pyruvic transaminase. Thirty percent of alcohol-dependent patients, compared with 1% of control subjects, have evidence of old rib fractures on chest x-ray.

Differential Diagnosis

The diagnosis of alcohol dependence is usually clear after careful history, physical and mental status examination, and consultation with family or friends.

Management

Management is specific to the clinical syndrome. Alcohol intoxication is treated with supportive measures, including decreasing external stimuli and withdrawing the source of alcohol. Intensive care may be required in cases of excessive alcohol intake complicated by respiratory compromise. All suspected or known alcohol-dependent patients should receive oral vitamin supplementation with folate 1 mg/day and thiamine 100 mg/day. If oral intake is not possible, thiamine should be injected intramuscularly before any glucose is given (because glucose depletes thiamine stores).

Alcohol withdrawal syndromes include the following.

Minor Withdrawal   *Chlordiazepoxide / Oxazepam.*

"The shakes" begin 12 to 18 hours after cessation of drinking and peak at 24 to 48 hours. Untreated, uncomplicated alcohol withdrawal lasts 5 to 7 days. It is characterized by tremors, nausea, vomiting, tachycardia, and hypertension. Minor withdrawal is treated with chlordiazepoxide (Librium) or oxazepam (Serax) titrated to the degree of withdrawal signs. The goals of treatment are prevention of more serious complications and patient comfort.

[margin handwriting, vertical: S E I Z U R E S H A L L U C I N. D E L I R I U M T R E M.]

Major Withdrawal

[handwriting above heading: seizures HALUS Delirium. ↓ ↓ ↓ BDZ, HALDOL BDZ+Supp.]

The risk of alcoholic seizures ("rum fits") begins 7 to 36 hours after cessation of drinking and peaks between **24 and 48 hours.** One to six generalized seizures are common but rarely lead to status epilepticus. Alcoholic seizures precede delirium tremens in 30% of cases. Seizures are treated acutely with intravenous **benzodiazepines.** Prophylactic phenytoin (Dilantin) should be administered during the high-risk period in patients with a history of withdrawal seizures.

Alcoholic hallucinosis has an onset within 48 hours of cessation of drinking and may last more than a week. It is characterized by vivid unpleasant auditory hallucinations in the presence of a clear sensorium. Alcoholic hallucinosis may be treated with a neuroleptic (e.g., haloperidol [Haldol] 2–5 mg twice a day). On rare occasions, these hallucinations become chronic.

Alcohol withdrawal delirium (delirium tremens) is a life-threatening condition manifested by delirium (perceptual disturbances, confusion or disorientation, agitation), autonomic hyperarousal, and mild fever. It affects up to 5% of hospitalized patients with alcohol dependence and typically begins 2 to 3 days after abrupt reduction in or cessation of alcohol intake. It is treated with intravenous benzodiazepines and supportive care. Treatment may need to occur in an intensive care unit, particularly if there is significant autonomic instability (e.g., rapidly fluctuating blood pressure). The syndrome typically lasts 3 days but can persist for weeks.

Alcohol Rehabilitation

The two goals of rehabilitation are **sobriety** and treatment of **comorbid psychopathology.**

To have a lasting recovery, the patient must stop denying the illness and accept the diagnosis of alcohol dependence. **Alcoholics Anonymous** (AA), a worldwide self-help group for recovering alcohol-dependent patients, has been shown to be one of the most effective programs for achieving and maintaining sobriety. The program involves daily to weekly meetings that focus on 12 steps toward recovery. Members are expected to pursue the 12 steps with the assistance of a sponsor (preferably someone with several years of sobriety).

Alcohol appears to be a potent depressant, so treatment of depression should be geared to patients who remain depressed after 2 to 4 weeks of sobriety. Anxiety is also common in withdrawing or newly sober patients and should be assessed after at least 1 month of sobriety.

Inpatient and residential rehabilitation programs use a team approach aimed at focusing the patient on recovery. Group therapy allows patients to see their own problems mirrored in and confronted by others. Family therapy allows the patient to examine the role of the family in alcoholism.

Disulfiram (Antabuse) can be helpful in maintaining sobriety in some patients. It acts by inhibiting the second enzyme in the pathway of alcohol metabolism, aldehyde dehydrogenase, so that acetaldehyde accumulates in the bloodstream, causing flushing, nausea, vomiting, palpitations, and hypotension. In theory, disulfiram should inhibit drinking by making it physiologically unpleasant; however, because the effects can be fatal in rare cases, patients must be committed to abstinence and fully understand the danger of drinking while taking disulfiram. The usual dose of disulfiram is 250 mg daily.

Many studies have demonstrated benefits from rehabilitation programs, but nearly half of all treated alcohol-dependent patients will relapse, most commonly in the first 6 months.

Key Points

In alcohol dependence,

1. Denial and minimization are common;
2. Withdrawal and delirium tremens are treated with benzodiazepines;
3. Peak incidence of alcoholic seizures is 24 to 48 hours; *[handwriting: also Hallucinosis DT = 2-3 days.]*
4. Rehabilitation is aimed at abstinence and treating comorbid disorders;
5. Rehabilitation involves AA and group and family therapies;
6. 50% of treated alcoholics will relapse.

In Wernicke-Korsakoff syndrome,

1. Wernicke-Korsakoff syndrome is due to thiamine deficiency;
2. Wernicke's triad is nystagmus, ataxia, and mental confusion;
3. Korsakoff's symptoms are anterograde amnesia and confabulation.

▶ SEDATIVE, HYPNOTIC, AND ANXIOLYTIC SUBSTANCE USE DISORDERS

Sedative, hypnotic, and anxiolytic drugs are widely used. They are all **cross-tolerant** with each other and with alcohol. Included in this class are barbiturates and benzodiazepines. Of these, the benzodiazepines are the most widely prescribed and available.

Epidemiology

Approximately 15% of the general population is prescribed a benzodiazepine in a given year. Some patients actually abuse these drugs.

Clinical Manifestations

History, Physical and Mental Status Examinations, and Laboratory Tests

Sedative-hypnotic drug abuse and dependence are associated with syndromes of intoxication, withdrawal, and withdrawal delirium that resemble those of alcohol.

Intoxication only can be distinguished from alcohol intoxication by the presence (or absence) of alcohol on the breath, serum, or urine. Barbiturates when taken orally are much more likely than benzodiazepines to cause clinically significant respiratory compromise. Intoxication can be confirmed through quantitative or qualitative serum or urine toxicologic analyses. Serum toxicologic screens can identify the presence of benzodiazepines and barbiturates and their major metabolites.

Withdrawal symptoms are listed in Table 5-1. Withdrawal delirium (confusion, disorientation, and visual and somatic hallucinations) has an onset of 3 to 4 days after abstinence. Dependence requires the presence of three or more of the seven maladaptive behaviors listed in Table 5-1.

Management

Treatment of sedative-hypnotic withdrawal may occur as an outpatient or on an inpatient unit. Generally, inpatient detoxification is required when there is comorbid medical or psychiatric illness, prior treatment failures, or when without support of family or friend.

TABLE 5-1
Sedative-Hypnotic Withdrawal

Minor Withdrawal	More Severe Withdrawal
Restlessness	Coarse tremors
Apprehension	Weakness
Anxiety	Vomiting
	Sweating
	Hyperreflexia
	Nausea
	Orthostatic hypotension
	Seizures

On an inpatient unit, benzodiazepines or barbiturates may be administered and tapered in a controlled manner. Withdrawal from short-acting substances is generally more **severe**, whereas withdrawal from longer-acting substances is more **prolonged**.

Withdrawal from barbiturates is more dangerous than benzodiazepines: it can (much more easily) lead to hyperpyrexia and death. Withdrawal is managed by scheduled dosing and tapering of a benzodiazepine or barbiturate (diazepam or phenobarbital).

In patients who have been abusing alcohol and benzodiazepines or barbiturates, it may be necessary to perform a **pentobarbital challenge test.** This test allows for the quantification of tolerance to perform a controlled taper, thereby reducing the problems of withdrawal.

Treatment of sedative-hypnotic dependence resembles that for alcohol dependence. After detoxification, the patient can enter a residential rehabilitation program or a day or evening treatment program. Referral to AA is appropriate because the addiction issues and recovery process are similar. Families may be referred to Al-Anon.

Key Points

Sedative-hypnotic drugs

1. Are cross-tolerant with alcohol;
2. Have intoxicating effects and withdrawal states similar to alcohol;
3. Tolerance can be measured by a pentobarbital challenge test;
4. Treatment resembles that for alcoholism.

▶ OPIOID USE DISORDERS

Opiates include morphine, heroin, codeine, meperidine, and hydromorphone. Heroin is only available illegally in the United States. Opiates are commonly used for pain control.

Epidemiology

Opiate use and abuse are relatively uncommon in the United States. Lifetime prevalence in 1991 was 0.9% and point prevalence was less than 0.1%. Many of those who use opiates recreationally become **addicted.** The number of opiate addicts in the United States is estimated at 500,000.

Clinical Manifestations

History, Physical and Mental Status Examinations, and Laboratory Tests

Most heroin and morphine users take opiates intravenously, which produces flushing and an intensely pleasurable diffuse bodily sensation that resembles orgasm. This initial "rush" is followed by a sense of well-being. Psychomotor retardation, drowsiness, inactivity, and impaired concentration ensue. Signs of intoxication occur immediately after the addict "shoots up" and include pupillary constriction, respiratory depression, slurred speech, hypotension, bradycardia, and hypothermia. Nausea, vomiting, and constipation are common after opiate use. Opiate use can be confirmed by urine or serum toxicologic measurements.

Opiate abuse is defined by the criteria for substance abuse noted above. In opiate dependence, tolerance to the effects of opiates occurs. Addicts "shoot up" three or more times per day.

Withdrawal symptoms usually begin 10 hours after the last dose. Withdrawal from opiates can be highly uncomfortable but is rarely medically complicated. Withdrawal symptoms are listed in Table 5-2.

Opiate addicts often have comorbid substance use disorders, antisocial or borderline personality disorders, and mood disorders. Opiate addicts are more prone to commit crimes because of the high cost of opiates. Opiate addiction also is associated with **high mortality rates** from **inadvertent overdoses, accidents,** and **suicide.** Opiate addicts are also at higher risk of medical problems because of poor nutrition and use of dirty needles. Common medical disorders include serum hepatitis, HIV infection, endocarditis, pneumonia, and cellulitis.

Differential Diagnosis

The diagnosis of opiate addiction is usually obvious after a careful history and mental status and physical examinations.

Management

Patients addicted to opiates should be gradually withdrawn using methadone. **Methadone** is a weak agonist of the *mu* opiate receptor and has a longer half-life (15 hours) than heroin or morphine. Thus, it causes relatively few intoxicant or withdrawal effects. Generally, the initial dose of methadone (typically 5–20 mg) is based on the profile of withdrawal symptoms. The dose is repeated as needed for the first 24 hours. The total 24-hour dose is then tapered by 5mg/day with a once per day administration schedule. Withdrawal from short-acting opiates lasts 7 to 10 days; withdrawal from longer-acting meperidine lasts 2 to 3 weeks.

Clonidine, a centrally acting alpha 2 receptor agonist that decreases central noradrenergic output, also,can be used for acute withdrawal syndromes. It is remarkably effective at treating the autonomic symptoms of withdrawal but does little to curb the drug craving. Risks of sedation and hypotension limit clonidine's usefulness in outpatient settings.

Rehabilitation generally involves referral to an intensive day treatment program and to Narcotics Anonymous, a 12-step program similar to AA. Methadone maintenance, daily administration of 60–100 mg of methadone in government-licensed methadone clinics, is used widely for patients with demonstrated physiologic dependence. Long-term administration of methadone can alleviate drug hunger and minimize drug-seeking behavior.

TABLE 5-2
Symptoms of Opiate Withdrawal ⟩Sympathetic + diarrhea

Mild Withdrawal

Dysphoric mood, anxiety, and restlessness

Lacrimation or rhinorrhea

Pupillary dilatation, piloerection, or sweating, hypertension and tachycardia   *Cold Turkey w/ Rapid HR*

Fever

Diarrhea

Insomnia

Yawning

More Severe Withdrawal

Nausea

Vomiting

Muscle aches

Seizures (in meperidine withdrawal)

Abdominal cramps

Hot and cold flashes

Severe anxiety

Key Points

1. Recreational use of opiates often leads to addiction;

2. Opiate addicts are at increased risk of HIV, pneumonia, endocarditis, hepatitis, and cellulitis;

3. High mortality occurs from accidental overdose, suicide, and accidents;

✳4. Opiate withdrawal begins 10 hours after last dose;

5. Withdrawal is uncomfortable but not usually medically complicated;

6. Withdrawal is treated with tapering doses of methadone; /+ clonidine

7. Methadone maintenance can be used successfully to reduce drug-seeking behavior.

► CENTRAL NERVOUS SYSTEM STIMULANT USE DISORDERS

Cocaine and amphetamines are readily available in the United States. The patterns of use, abuse, and dependence of cocaine and amphetamines are similar because both are central nervous stimulants with similar psychoactive and sympathomimetic effects.

In the United States, cocaine is available in two forms: cocaine hydrochloride powder, which is typically snorted, and cocaine alkaloid crystal ("crack"), which is typically smoked. Cocaine has an extremely rapid onset of action (when snorted or smoked) and a short half-life, requiring frequent dosing to remain "high."

In the United States, amphetamines (amphetamine, dextroamphetamine, and methamphetamine) are available in pill form by prescription for the treatment of obesity, narcolepsy, and attention deficit/hyperactivity disorder. A very pure form of methamphetamine, called crystal methamphetamine, can be snorted; it is available illegally in the United States and is smoked. Amphetamines have a longer half-life than cocaine and hence are self-administered less frequently.

Clinical Manifestations

Cocaine or amphetamine intoxication is characterized by

1. Maladaptive behavioral changes (e.g., euphoria or hypervigilance);
2. Tachycardia or bradycardia;
3. Pupillary dilatation;
4. Hyper- or hypotension;
5. Perspiration or chills;
6. Nausea or vomiting;

Sympathetic Activation + Resp. Depression

7. Weight loss;
8. Psychomotor agitation or retardation;
9. Muscular weakness, respiratory depression, chest pain, cardiac dysrhythmias;
10. Confusion, seizures, dyskinesia, or coma.

Cocaine intoxication can cause tactile hallucinations ("coke bugs"). Both cocaine and amphetamine intoxication can lead to agitation, impaired judgment, and **transient psychosis** (e.g., paranoia, visual hallucinations). Cocaine and amphetamine dependence is defined by the criteria outlined above for substance dependence.

Withdrawal of cocaine or amphetamines leads to fatigue, depression, nightmares, headache, profuse sweating, muscle cramps, and hunger. Withdrawal symptoms peak in **2 to 4 days.**

Management

Withdrawal from amphetamines or other central nervous system stimulants is **self-limited** and usually does not require inpatient detoxification. Psychosis from amphetamine intoxication or withdrawal is generally self-limited, requiring only observation in a safe environment. Antipsychotic medications can be used for agitation.

Ultimately, the goal is rehabilitation. Narcotics Anonymous, treatment of comorbid psychopathology, drugs to reduce craving, and family therapy are the essential features of cocaine rehabilitation.

Key Points

1. Cocaine and amphetamines are CNS stimulants;
2. CNS stimulants can cause transient psychosis (e.g., "coke bugs" or paranoia); + Visual Hallucinations
3. Withdrawal symptoms of CNS stimulants (fatigue, depression, nightmares, etc.) peak in 2 to 4 days.
4. Withdrawal from CNS stimulants is self-limited.

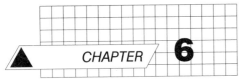

CHAPTER 6

Eating Disorders

$\mathcal{E}$ating disorders are characterized by disturbances in eating behavior and an overconcern with body image or size. Although eating disorders are classified into two discrete diagnostic categories in the *Diagnostic and Statistical Manual of Mental Disorders*, 4th edition (DSM-IV), many symptoms overlap. The principal diagnostic distinction is based on ideal body weight. When abnormal eating behavior causes body weight to fall below a defined percentage of expected body weight, a diagnosis of anorexia nervosa is made. If ideal body weight is maintained in the presence of abnormal eating behaviors, a diagnosis of bulimia nervosa is made. Eating disorders likely lie along a continuum of disturbances in eating behavior and often are associated with mood disorders and other psychiatric illnesses (Table 6-1).

▶ ANOREXIA NERVOSA

Anorexia nervosa is a severe eating disorder characterized by **low body weight**. Anorexia nervosa is diagnosed when a person's body weight falls below 15% of the ideal weight for that individual. The weight loss must be due to behavior directed at maintaining low weight or achieving a particular body image.

Epidemiology

The point prevalence of anorexia nervosa is between 0.5% and 1% in women, and over 90% of patients with anorexia nervosa are women. The prevalence in men is not clear. Average age of onset is 17; onset is rare before puberty or after age 40. Anorexia nervosa is more common in industrial societies and higher socioeconomic classes.

Etiology

Eating disorders and their subtypes likely share many common bases of origin. Psychological theories of an-

orexia nervosa remain speculative. Patients with anorexia nervosa generally have a high fear of losing control, difficulty with self-esteem, and commonly display "all or none" thinking. Although it is not specific to eating disorders, past physical or sexual abuse may be a risk factor. Contemporary theories focus on the need to control one's body.

Social theories propose that societal opinions, which equate low body weight with attractiveness, drive women to develop eating disorders. Although this fact may be responsible for some cases (e.g., anorexia nervosa is more common among dancers and models), historically anorexia nervosa has been present during periods when societal mores for beauty were different.

Biologic, familial, and genetic data support a biologic and heritable basis for anorexia. Family studies reveal an increased incidence of mood disorders and anorexia nervosa in first-degree relatives of patients with anorexia nervosa. Twin studies show higher concordance for monozygotic versus dizygotic twin pairs. Neuroendocrine evidence supporting a biologic contribution to anorexia includes alterations in corticotropin-releasing factor, reduced central nervous system norepinephrine metabolism, and that amenorrhea (caused by decreased luteinizing hormone and follicle-stimulating hormone release) sometimes precedes the onset of anorexia nervosa.

Clinical Manifestations

History and Mental Status Examination

DSM-IV criteria for the diagnosis of anorexia nervosa include refusal to keep body weight at greater than 85% of ideal, an intense fear of weight gain, preoccupation with body size and shape, a disproportionate influence of body weight on personal worth, and the denial of the medical risks of low weight. Patients with anorexia nervosa generally do not have a loss of appetite; they refuse to eat out of fear of gaining weight. Amenorrhea is also a diagnostic criteria in postmenarchal females (delay of menarche may occur in premenarchal girls). In some cases, amenorrhea precedes the development of anorexia nervosa; however, in most cases it appears to be a consequence of starvation.

TABLE 6-1

Classification of Eating Disorders

Anorexia Nervosa	Bulimia Nervosa
Restricting type	Nonpurging type
Binge eating/purging type	Purging type

Individuals with anorexia nervosa commonly exercise intensely to lose weight and alter their body shape. Some restrict food intake as a primary method of weight control; others use binging and purging (use of laxatives, enemas, diuretics, or induced vomiting) to control weight.

The behavioral repertoire used to control body weight is used to further classify anorexia nervosa into two subtypes: restricting type and binging/purging type. In the restricting type, the major methods of weight control are food restriction and exercise. In the binging/purging type, food restriction and exercise also may be present, but binge eating and subsequent purging behaviors also are present.

The natural course of anorexia is not well understood, but many cases become chronic. The long-term mortality of anorexia nervosa secondary to suicide or medical complications is greater than 10%.

Differential Diagnosis

Conditions that can resemble anorexia should be ruled out. These include major depression with loss of appetite and weight, some psychotic disorders where nutrition may not be adequate, body dysmorphic disorder, and a variety of general medical (especially neuroendocrine) conditions. Anorexia nervosa is differentiated from bulimia nervosa by the presence of low weight in the former.

Management

The management of anorexia nervosa is directed at the presenting symptoms. When medical complications are present, these must be carefully treated and followed. If ipecac use to induce vomiting is suspected, ipecac toxicity must be ruled out.

During starvation, psychotherapy is of little value because of the cognitive impairment produced by starvation. When patients are less medically ill, a therapeutic program, including supervised meals, weight and electrolyte monitoring, psychoeducation about the illness, starvation, nutrition, individual psychotherapy, and family therapy, are all used. Psychopharmacology management often includes antidepressants, especially the selective serotonin reuptake inhibitors (SSRIs) to treat comorbid depression. Psychopharmacologic treatments are used principally to treat any comorbid psychiatric illness and have little or no effect on the anorexia per se.

Key Points

Anorexia nervosa

1. Is a severe eating disorder characterized by low body weight;

2. Is diagnosed over 90% of the time in women;

3. Has serious medical complications;

4. Has a greater than 10% long-term mortality rate.

▶ BULIMIA NERVOSA

Bulimia nervosa is an eating disorder characterized by **binge eating** with the **maintenance of body weight.**

Epidemiology

The estimated point prevalence of bulimia nervosa is 1% to 3% of women. The male-to-female ratio is 1:10. This illness occurs disproportionately among whites in the United States.

Etiology

Many of the factors in the genesis of anorexia nervosa also are implicated in bulimia nervosa. Familial and genetic studies support similar familial linkages in both disorders. Psychological theories for bulimia nervosa stress an addiction or obsessive/compulsive behavioral model. Biologic, neurologic, and endocrine findings are less prominent in theories of causation of bulimia nervosa. Abnormal serotonin metabolism also is thought to play more of a role in bulimia nervosa than in anorexia nervosa.

Clinical Manifestations

History and Mental Status Examination

Bulimia nervosa is diagnosed in individuals who have binge eating and behaviors designed to avoid weight gain but who maintain their body weight. In addition, these are people whose self-evaluation is overly influenced by their body weight and shape.

Food binges in bulimia nervosa may be precipitated by stress or altered mood states. Once a binge begins, the individual typically feels out of control and continues to eat large quantities of food, often to the point of physical discomfort. **Purging** may follow and most often consists of vomiting, usually induced mechanically by stimulating the gag reflex; ipecac sometimes is used. Other purging methods used to avoid weight gain include laxative and diuretic abuse and enemas. Bulimic individuals often exercise and restrict their food intake. As in anorexia nervosa, patients with bulimia nervosa are overconcerned with body image and have a preoccupation with becoming fat. Bulimia nervosa is classified into two subtypes: nonpurging type or **purging** type (see Table 6-1) according to whether **purging** behavior is present.

Differential Diagnosis

Bulimia nervosa should be distinguished from the binge eating and purging subtype of anorexia nervosa. If body weight is less than 15% of ideal, a diagnosis of anorexia nervosa is made. Binge eating can occur in major depression and in borderline personality disorder but is not tied to a compulsion to reduce weight.

Management

The treatment for bulimia nervosa is similar to that for anorexia nervosa. Although medical complications of starvation are not present, other medical complications can require careful medical management and, at times, hospitalization. Psychotherapy focuses at first on achieving behavioral control of eating behavior. Cognitive therapy may be useful in treating overconcern with body image. Self-esteem and interpersonal relationships become the focus of therapy as the behavioral dyscontrol abates. Antidepressants, especially SSRIs, are more effective in the treatment of bulimia nervosa than in anorexia nervosa (including those patients who do not have comorbid depression).

Key Points

Bulimia nervosa

1. Is a severe eating disorder characterized by binge eating and purging;

2. Is also characterized by maintenance of normal bodyweight;

3. Is more common in women than in men;

4. Can have serious medical complications.

5. Better Response to SSRI's.

▶ MEDICAL COMPLICATIONS)

Eating disorders, when persistent, can have serious medical consequences. The lifetime mortality from anorexia nervosa is approximately 10%; it is unknown for bulimia nervosa. Table 6-2 lists the common medical complications of eating disorders. The most serious of these, gastricoresophageal rupture, cardiomyopathy

TABLE 6-2

Medical Complications of Eating Disorders

Behavior	Medical Complication
Binge eating	Gastric dilatation or rupture
Vomiting	Esophageal rupture
	Parotiditis with hyperamylassemia
	Hypokalemic, hypochloremic, metabolic alkalosis (with cardiac arrhythmias)
	Ipecactoxicity (cardiac and skeletal myopathies)
Laxative use	Constipation (due to laxative dependence)
	Metabolic acidosis
	Dehydration
Diuretic use	Electrolyte abnormalities (with cardiac arrhythmias)
	Dehydration
Starvation	Leukopenia, anemia
	Increased ventricular/brain ratio
	Hypotension, bradycardia
	Hypothermia
	Hypercholesterolemia
	Edema
	Dryskin, lanugo hair

from ipecactoxicity, and cardiac arrhythmias secondary to electrolyte imbalance, can be fatal. Other complications parallel those of chronic medical illness, take a severe toll on the patient's overall functioning, and cause tremendous suffering and burden to their families. In addition to these medical complications, secondary psychiatric and neurologic sequela include cognitive decline, metabolic encephalopathy, and severe mood disturbance, all with profound consequences to patients and their families.

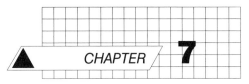

CHAPTER 7

Disorders of Childhood and Adolescence

*M*any disorders seen in adults can occur in children. There are, however, a group of disorders usually first diagnosed in children and hence bear specifically on children. These disorders of childhood and adolescence are listed in Table 7-1.

Child psychiatric assessment requires attention to details of a child's stage of development, family structure and dynamics, and normative age-appropriate behavior. Consultation with parents and obtaining information from schools, teachers, and other involved parties (e.g., Department of Social Services/Youth Services) is essential to proper assessment.

Children, especially young children, usually express emotion in a more **concrete** (less abstract) way than adults. Consequently, child interviews require more concrete queries (Do you feel like crying? *instead of* Are you sad?). Playing games, taking turns telling stories, and imaginative play often are used to gain insight into the child's emotional and interpersonal life. During play, observations also are made regarding activity level, motor skills, and verbal expression. Children are much more likely than adults to have **comorbid** mental disorders, making diagnosis and treatment more complicated.

The complexities of diagnosis in child psychiatry often require the use of psychological testing. Tests of **General Intelligence** include the Stanford-Binet Intelligence Scale (one of the first IQ tests developed and often used in young children) and the Wechsler Intelligence Scale for Children-Revised (WISC-R). The WISC-R is the most widely used intelligence test for assessing school-age children. It yields a verbal score, a performance score, and a full-scale score (both verbal and performance) or **intelligence quotient (IQ)**.

TABLE 7-1
Common Psychiatric Disorders of Childhood and Adolescence

Mental retardation	Attention-deficit/
Learning disorders	hyperactivity disorder
Communication disorders	Conduct disorder/
Autistic disorder	oppositional defiant
	Tourette's disorder
	Separation anxiety disorder

TABLE 7-2		
Mental Retardation		
Degree of MR	IQ	Percentage of Total MR Population
Mild	50–70	85%
Moderate	35–50	10%
Severe	20–35	3–4%
Profound	< 20	1–2%

There are many other tests and objective rating scales designed to measure behavior (e.g., impulsiveness, physical activity), perceptual-motor skills (by drawing people, placing pegs in appropriately shaped holes), and personality style (by describing what is happening in an ambiguous scene).

Because seizure activity or subtle electroencephalographic abnormalities are common in certain child psychiatric disorders, an **electroencephalogram (EEG)** may be warranted. The evaluation of mental retardation usually involves a search for possible causes. **Karyotyping** may be used to identify Fragile X syndrome, Down syndrome, or XYY.

▶ MENTAL RETARDATION

Patients with mental retardation have subnormal intelligence (as measured by IQ) combined with deficits in adaptive functioning. IQ is defined as the mental age (as assessed using a WISC-R) divided by the chronologic age and multiplied by 100. If mental age equals chronologic age, then the ratio equals one and the IQ is "100." An IQ of **less than** 70 is required for the diagnosis of mental retardation. Severity ranges from mild to profound and is based on IQ (Table 7-2).

Epidemiology *male > female*

Mental retardation affects 1% to 2% of the population and has a male-to-female ratio of **2:1.** Milder forms of mental retardation occur more frequently in families with low socioeconomic status (SES); more severe forms of mental retardation are independent of SES. Most patients with mental retardation have mild or moderate forms (see Table 7-2).

Etiology

Mental retardation can be thought of as a final common pathway of a number of childhood or perinatal disorders. The most common cause of mental retardation is **Down syndrome** (trisomy 21). Fragile X syndrome is the most common cause of heritable mental retardation. Inborn errors of metabolism, perinatal or early childhood head injuries, maternal diabetes, substance abuse, toxemia, or rubella can all cause mental retardation. Overall, there are more than 500 genetic abnormalities associated with mental retardation.

Clinical Manifestations

History, Physical and Mental Status Examinations, and Laboratory Tests

Most mentally retarded children have physical malformations that identify them at birth as high risk for mental retardation (such as the characteristic facies of the child with Down syndrome). Infants can show signs of significantly subaverage intellectual functioning. Young children with mental retardation may be identified by parents or pediatricians after failure to meet developmental milestones in a number of functional areas (e.g., delayed speech, social skills, or self-care skills capacity) or on scoring an IQ less than 70 on the Stanford-Binet (usually only for very young children) or WISC-R (standard for school-age children).

The onset of symptoms must be before age 18. The patient must have both an IQ less than or equal to 70 and concurrent deficits or impairments in several areas of adaptive functioning (e.g., communication, self-care, interpersonal skills).

Differential Diagnosis

Attention-deficit/hyperactivity disorder, learning disorders, depression, schizophrenia, and seizure disorder can all resemble mental retardation. These disorders also can be comorbid conditions. Children suspected of having mental retardation should have a thorough medical and neurologic evaluation, including IQ testing, an EEG, and brain imaging (CT or MRI).

Management

Management depends on the degree of retardation, the course, and the particular abilities of the child and their parents. Most children with mental retardation progress through normal milestones (standing, walking, talking, learning to recognize letters and numbers) in a similar pattern to normal children **but at a slower rate**. Growth and development occur in chil-

dren with mental retardation. They can have developmental spurts, like normal children, that could not have been predicted at an earlier age.

In mild mental retardation, the child is typically considered educable. The child usually can learn to read, write, and perform simple arithmetic. With family support and special education, most of these children will be able to live with their parents. The long-term goal of treatment is to function in the community and to hold some type of job.

In moderate mental retardation, the child is typically considered trainable. With training, they can learn to talk, recognize their name and a few simple words, and perform activities of daily living (bathing, dressing, handling small change) without assistance. The long-term goal of treatment typically is shelter in a supervised group home.

Children with severe or profound mental retardation almost invariably require care in institutional settings, usually beginning very early in life. These forms of mental retardation often are associated with specific syndromes (e.g., Tay-Sachs disease) in which there is progressive physical deterioration leading to premature death.

Key Points

Mental retardation is

1. Defined by IQ less than or equal to 70 and functioning in specific areas;

2. More common in males (2:1);

3. Most commonly caused by Down syndrome (trisomy 21); *Heritable #1 is Fragile X.*

4. Managed in developmentally appropriate settings.

▶ LEARNING DISORDERS

Learning disorders are characterized by performance in a specific area of learning (e.g., reading, writing, arithmetic) substantially below the expectation of a child's chronologic age, measured intelligence, and age-appropriate education. The *Diagnostic and Statistical Manual of Mental Disorders*, 4th edition, identifies three learning disorders: **reading disorder, mathematics disorder,** and **disorder of written expression.**

Etiology

Specific learning disorders often occur in **families.** They are presumed to result from **focal cerebral injury** or from a **neurodevelopmental defect.**

Epidemiology _Male > Female_

Learning disorders are relatively common. Reading disorder affects 4% of school-age children and mathematics disorder is estimated at 1%. The incidence of disorder of written expression is not yet known. Learning disorders are **two to four times** more common in boys than girls.

Clinical Manifestations

History, Mental Status Examination, and Laboratory Tests _Higher IQ then Achievements Show._

Patients with specific learning disorders are typically diagnosed after the child has exhibited difficulties in a specific academic area. Because reading and arithmetic are usually not taught before the first grade, the diagnosis is seldom made in preschoolers. Some children may not be diagnosed until fourth or fifth grade, particularly if they have a high IQ and can mask their specific deficit. The diagnosis of learning disorder is confirmed through specific **intelligence** and **achievement testing.** Children with <u>learning disorder</u> do not obtain achievement test scores consistent with their overall IQ.

Differential Diagnosis

It is important to establish that a low achievement score is not due to some other factor such as lack of opportunity to learn, poor teaching, or cultural factors (e.g., English as a second language). Physical factors (such as hearing or vision impairment) also must be ruled out.

Finally, it is important to consider and test for more global disorders such as pervasive developmental disorder, mental retardation, and communication disorders. It is not uncommon to find many of these disorders coexist. A specific learning disorder diagnosis is made when the full clinical picture is not adequately explained by other comorbid conditions.

Management

Children with these disorders often need **remedial education,** especially if their diagnosis was made late. They also need to be taught **learning strategies** to overcome their particular deficit(s). Acceptable skills in the disordered area often can be achieved with steady supportive educational assistance.

Key Points

In learning disorders,

1. There are three types: mathematics, reading, and written expression;

2. They are familial and probably due to cerebral injury or maldevelopment;

3. Reading disorder is most common and all three disorders occur more in boys (2 to 4:1);

4. The diagnosis is confirmed through achievement tests;

5. Physical or social factors must be ruled out;

6. Management involves remedial education and learning strategies.

▶ AUTISTIC DISORDER

Autistic disorder is the most common of the pervasive developmental disorders of childhood onset. It is characterized by the triad of impaired social interactions, impaired ability to communicate, and restricted repertoire of activities and interests.

Etiology

Autistic disorder is **familial.** Genetic studies demonstrate incomplete penetrance (36% concordance rate in monozygotic twins), although a specific genetic defect has not been discovered. A small percentage of those with autistic disorder have a **fragile X** chromosome, and a high rate of autism exists with **tuberous sclerosis.**

Epidemiology

Autistic disorder is rare. It occurs in two to five children per 10,000 live births. The male to female sex ratio is 3 to 4:1.

Clinical Manifestations

History, Mental Status Examination, and Laboratory Tests

Abnormal development usually is first noted soon after birth. Commonly, the first sign is **impairment in social interactions** (failure to develop a <u>social smile,</u> facial expressions, or <u>eye-to-eye gaze</u>). Older children often fail to develop nonverbal forms of communication (e.g., body postures and gestures) and may seem to have no desire or lack the skills to form friendships. There is also a lack of seeking to share enjoyment (i.e., not showing, sharing, or pointing out objects they find interesting).

Autistic disorder is also characterized by a **marked impairment in communication.** There may be delay in or total lack of language development. Those children who do develop language show impairment in the ability to initiate and sustain conversations and the use of repetitive or idiosyncratic language. Language also may be abnormal in pitch, intonation, rate, rhythm, or stress.

Finally, there are usually **restrictive, repetitive,** or **stereotyped patterns** of **behavior, interests,** or **activities.** There may be an encompassing preoccupation with one or more stereotyped and restricted patterns of interest (e.g., amassing baseball trivia), an inflexible adherence to specific nonfunctional routines or rituals (e.g., eating the same meal in the same place at the same time each day), stereotyped or repetitive motor mannerisms (e.g., whole-body rocking), and a persistent preoccupation with the parts of objects (e.g., buttons).

Approximately **25%** of children with autistic disorder have comorbid seizures; approximately **75%** have mental retardation (the moderate type is most common). [35-50 Score.] EEGs and intelligence testing typically are part of the initial evaluation.

Differential Diagnosis

The diagnosis is usually clear after careful history, mental status examination, and developmental monitoring. However, childhood psychosis, mental retardation (alone), language disorders, and congenital deafness or blindness must all be ruled out.

Management

Autistic disorder is a chronic life-long disorder with relatively severe morbidity. Very few individuals with autism will ever live independently. Once the diagnosis is made, parents should be informed that their child has a neurodevelopmental disorder (not a behavioral disorder that they might feel responsible for creating). They will have to learn **behavioral management techniques** designed to reduce the rigid and stereotyped behaviors of the disorder as well as how to improve social functioning. Many children with autism require special education or specialized day programs for behavior management.

Autistic children with a comorbid seizure disorder are treated with anticonvulsants. Low doses of **neuroleptics** (e.g., haloperidol) and some mood stabilizers and antidepressants have been shown to help decrease aggressive or self-harming behaviors.

Key Points

Autistic disorder

1. Is a rare pervasive developmental disorder characterized by impaired social interactions, impaired ability to communicate, and restricted repertoire of activities and interests;

2. Is familial and associated with fragile X syndrome and tuberous sclerosis;

3. Has a comorbid seizure rate of 25%;

4. Has a mental retardation rate of 75%;

5. Is managed by behavioral techniques and neuroleptics. + Anticonvulsants.

▶ ATTENTION DEFICIT/HYPERACTIVITY DISORDER

Attention Deficit/Hyperactivity Disorder (ADHD) is characterized by a persistent and dysfunctional pattern of overactivity, impulsiveness, inattention, and distractibility.

Etiology

The disorder runs in families and also cosegregates with mood disorders, substance use disorders, learning disorders, and antisocial personality disorder. Families with a child diagnosed with ADHD are more likely than those without ADHD offspring to have family members with the above-mentioned disorders.

The etiology of the disorder is unknown, but perinatal injury, malnutrition, and substance exposure all have been implicated. Many children with ADHD have abnormalities of sleep architecture (decreased rapid eye movement latency, increased delta latency), EEG, and soft neurologic signs.

Epidemiology

The prevalence of ADHD in school-age children is estimated to be 3% to 5%. The sex ratio ranges from **4:1** in the general population to **9:1** in clinical settings. Boys are much more likely than girls to be brought to medical attention.

Clinical Manifestations

History, Mental Status Examination, and Laboratory Tests

To meet criteria for ADHD, a child must have evidence of the onset of **inattentive** or **hyperactive** symptoms before age 7; symptoms also must be present in two or more settings (e.g., school, home). Symptoms in only one setting suggest an environmental or psychodynamic cause.

Preschool-age children usually are brought for evaluation when unmanageable at home. Typically, they stay up late, wake up early, and spend most of their waking hours in many types of hyperactive and impulsive activities. Children with a great deal of hyperactivity may literally run about the house, cause damage, and wreak havoc.

When these children enter school, their difficulties with attention become more obvious. They appear to not follow directions, forget important school supplies, fail to complete homework or in-class assignments, and attempt to blurt out answers to teacher's questions before being called on. As a result of their inattention and hyperactivity, these children often become known as "troublemakers." They fall behind their peers academically and socially.

Evaluation of the child involves careful history gathering from parents and teachers (the latter usually through report cards and written reports). The child's behavior with and without the parent is carefully observed during psychiatric assessment. Informal testing is carried out by having the child attempt to complete a simple puzzle, write the letters of the alphabet, distinguish right and left, and recognize letters traced on his palms (graphesthesia). Physical examination, particularly focusing on neurologic function, is imperative. There are no specific laboratory or cognitive tests that are helpful in making the diagnosis.

Differential Diagnosis

It is important to distinguish symptoms of ADHD from age-appropriate behaviors in active children (running about, being noisy, etc.). Children also can appear inattentive if they have a low or a high IQ when the environment is overstimulating or understimulating, respectively. In either instance, IQ testing and careful evaluation of the school program will clarify the diagnosis.

Children with oppositional defiant disorder may resist work or school tasks because of an unwillingness to comply with others demands but not out of difficulty in attention.

Children with other mental disorders (e.g., mood disorder, anxiety disorder) can exhibit inattention but typically not before age 7. The child's history of school adjustment is not usually characterized by teacher or parent reports of inattentive disruptive behavior.

Symptoms that resemble ADHD can occur in children before age 7, but the etiology is typically a side effect of a medication (e.g., bronchodilators) or a psychotic or pervasive developmental disorder; these children are not considered to have ADHD. Of course, ADHD may be comorbid with any of the above disorders. A dual diagnosis is made only when it is needed to explain the full clinical picture.

Management

The management of ADHD involves a combination of somatic and behavioral treatments. Most children with ADHD respond favorably to **psychostimulants.** Methylphenidate is the first-line agent, followed by D-amphetamine. Clinicians try to use the smallest effective dose and to restrict use to periods of greatest need (i.e., the school day) because psychostimulants have undesirable long-term physical effects (weight gain and inhibited body growth).

Behavioral management techniques include positive reinforcement, firm limit-setting, and techniques for reducing stimulation (e.g., one playmate at a time, short, focused tasks).

Key Points

Attention deficit/hyperactivity disorder

1. Is characterized by inattentiveness and hyperactivity, occurring in multiple settings;

2. Symptoms must begin before age 7;

3. Is more common in boys (4:1);

4. Must rule out other causes of inattentiveness or hyperactivity;

5. Is managed with psychostimulants and behavioral techniques. *Methylphenidate, D-Ampletamine.*

▶ CONDUCT DISORDER AND OPPOSITIONAL DEFIANT DISORDER

Conduct disorder is defined as a repetitive and persistent pattern of behavior in which the basic rights of others or important age-appropriate societal norms or rules are violated. Disordered behaviors include aggression to people or animals, destruction of property, deceitfulness, theft, or serious violations of rules (school truancy, running away). Conduct disorder is the childhood equivalent of adult antisocial personality disorder. It is the most common diagnosis seen in outpatient psychiatric clinics and is frequently seen comorbidly with ADHD or learning disorders. Adoption studies show a genetic predisposition, but psychosocial factors play a major role. Parental separation or divorce, parental substance abuse, severely poor or inconsistent parenting, and association with a delinquent peer group have been shown to have some relationship to the development of conduct disorder.

Treatment involves individual and family therapy. Some children may need to be removed from the home and placed in foster care. Parents who retain custody of a child with conduct disorder are taught limit setting, consistency, and other behavioral techniques. Medications are used only to treat a comorbid ADHD or mood disorder but not for the conduct disorder itself. The long-term outcome depends on the severity of the disorder and the degree and type of comorbidity. Twenty-five percent to 40% of children with conduct disorder go on to have adult antisocial personality disorder.

Oppositional defiant disorder is diagnosed in children with annoying, difficult, or disruptive behavior when the frequency of the behavior significantly exceeds other children of his or her mental age (or that is less tolerated in the child's particular culture). It is a relatively new diagnosis that is meant to describe children with behavior problems that do not meet criteria for full-blown conduct disorder. Management emphasizes individual and family counseling.

Key Points

Conduct disorder

1. Is the childhood equivalent of antisocial personality disorder;
2. Is defined by observable measurable behaviors;
*3. Is the most common diagnosis in outpatient child psychiatric clinics;
4. Is managed by limit-setting, consistency, and behavioral techniques.

Oppositional defiant disorder

1. Is a less severe form of conduct disorder.

▶ TOURETTE'S DISORDER

Tourette's disorder is a rare disorder in which the child demonstrates multiple involuntary motor and vocal tics. A tic is a sudden, rapid, recurrent, nonrhythmic, stereotyped motor movement or vocalization.

Epidemiology   male > fem.

Tourette's disorder affects **0.4%** of the population. There is a **3:1** male-female ratio.

Etiology

Tourette's disorder is highly familial and appears to co-occur frequently with obsessive-compulsive disorder. Despite evidence of genetic transmission in some families, no gene (or genes) has yet been discovered to explain the etiology of the disorder.

Clinical Manifestations

History, Mental Status and Physical Examinations

The patient or family usually describes an onset in childhood or early adolescence before age 18. Vocal tics are usually loud grunts or barks but can involve shouting words; the words are sometimes obscenities (coprolalia). The patient describes being aware of shouting the words, being able to exert some control over them, but being overwhelmed by an uncontrollable urge to say them. Motor tics can involve facial grimacing, tongue protrusion, blinking, snorting, or larger movements of the extremities or whole body. Motor tics typically antedate vocal tics; barks or grunts typically antedate verbal shouts.

Differential Diagnosis

A careful neurologic evaluation should be performed to rule out other causes of tics. Wilson's disease and Huntington's disease are the principal differential diagnostic disorders. An EEG should be performed to rule out a seizure disorder. Careful evaluation for other comorbid psychiatric illnesses should be performed.

Management

Treatment typically involves the use of low doses of **high-potency neuroleptics** such as haloperidol or pimozide. The child and his or her family should receive education and **supportive psychotherapy** aimed at minimizing the negative social consequences (e.g., embarrassment, shame, isolation) that occur with this disorder.

Key Points

Tourette's disorder

1. Is a tic disorder;
2. Is rare and more common in males (3:1);
3. Must rule out Wilson's and Huntington's diseases;
4. Is treated with high-potency neuroleptics and patient/family support.

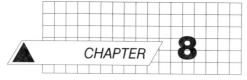

CHAPTER 8

Cognitive Disorders

The cognitive disorders are delirium, dementia, and amnestic disorders. Table 8-1 lists the *Diagnostic and Statistical Manual of Mental Disorders*, 4th edition, classification of cognitive disorders.

▶ DELIRIUM

Delirium is a reversible state of global cortical dysfunction characterized by alterations in **attention** and **cognition** and produced by a definable precipitant. Delirium is categorized by its etiology (see Table 8-1) as due to general medical conditions, as substance related, or multifactorial in origin.

Etiology

Delirium is a syndrome with many different causes. Most frequently, delirium is the result of a general medical condition; substance intoxication and withdrawal also are common causes. Structural central nervous system lesions also can lead to delirium. Table 8-2 lists common general medical and substance-related causes of delirium. Delirium is often multifactorial and may be produced by a combination of minor illnesses and minor metabolic derangements (e.g., mild anemia, mild hyponatremia, mild hypoxia, and urinary tract infection, especially in an elderly person).

TABLE 8-1

Cognitive Disorders

Delirium	Dementia	Amnestic
General medical	Alzheimer's type	General medical
Substance related	Vascular origin	Substance related
Multifactorial	HIV related	
	Head trauma related	
	Parkinson's related	
	Huntington's related	
	Pick's related	
	Creutzfeldt-Jakob related	
	General medical origin	
	Substance related	
	Multiple etiologies	

TABLE 8-2

Common Causes of Delirium

General Medical	Substance Related
Infectious	Intoxication
✱Urinary tract infections	Alcohol
Meningitis	Hallucinogens
Sepsis	Opioids
Metabolic	Marijuana
Hyponatremia	Stimulants
Hepatic encephalopathy	Sedatives
Hypoxia	Withdrawal
Hypercarbia	Alcohol
Hypoglycemia	Benzodiazepines
Fluid imbalance	Barbiturates
Uremia	Medication induced
Hypercalcemia	Anesthetics
Postsurgical	→ Anticholinergics
Hyper/hypothyroidism	Meperidine
Ictal/postictal	Antibiotics
Head trauma	Toxins
Miscellaneous	Carbon monoxide
Fat emboli syndrome	Organophosphates
Thiamine deficiency	↳ AChE Inhibitors.
Anemia	

Common medical causes of delirium include metabolic abnormalities such as hyponatremia, hypoxia, hypercapnia, hypoglycemia, and hypercalcemia: infectious illnesses, especially urinary tract infections, pneumonia, and meningitis, are often implicated. The common substance-induced causes of delirium are alcohol or benzodiazepine <u>withdrawal</u> and benzodiazepine and anticholinergic drug toxicity, although a great number of commonly used medications, prescribed and over the counter, can produce delirium. Other conditions predisposing to delirium include old age, fractures, and pre-existing dementia.

Epidemiology

The exact prevalence in the general population is unknown. Delirium occurs in 10% to 15% of general medical patients over age 65 and is seen frequently postsurgically and in intensive care units. Delirium is equally common in males and females.

Clinical Manifestations

History and Mental Status Examination

History is critical in the diagnosis of delirium, particularly in regard to the time course of development of the delirium and to the prior existence of dementia or other psychiatric illness. Key features of delirium are

1. Disturbance of consciousness, especially attention and level of arousal;

2. Alterations in cognition, especially memory, orientation, language, and perception;

3. Development over a period of hours to days;

4. Presence of medical or substance-related precipitants.

In addition, sleep-wake cycle disturbances and psychomotor agitation may occur. Delirium often is difficult to separate from dementia, in part because dementia is a risk factor for delirium (and thus they frequently co-occur) and in part because there is a great deal of symptom overlap, as outlined in Table 8-3. Key differentiating factors are the **time course** of development of the mental status change (especially if the patient did not have a prior dementia) and the presence of a **likely precipitant** for the mental status change. Individuals with delirium also may display periods of complete lucidity interspersed with periods of confusion, whereas in dementia the deficits are generally more stable. In both conditions, there may be nocturnal worsening of symptoms with increased agitation and confusion ("sundowning").

The diagnosis of delirium is complicated by the fact that there are no definitive tests for delirium. The workup for delirium includes a thorough history and mental status examination, a physical examination, and laboratory tests targeted at identifying general medical and substance related causes. These should include urinalysis, complete chemistry panel, complete blood count, and oxygen saturation. Additional workup might entail chest x-ray, arterial blood gas (ABG), neuroimaging, or electroencephalogram (EEG). EEG may reveal nonspecific diffuse slowing. The presence of a delirium is associated with a **1-year mortality rate of 40% to 50%.**

Differential Diagnosis

Delirium should be differentiated from dementia (although both can be present at the same time), psychotic or manic disorganization, and status complex partial epilepsy.

Management

The treatment of delirium involves keeping the patient safe from harm while addressing the delirium. In the case of delirium due to a general medical illness, the underlying illness must be treated; in substance-related delirium, treatment involves removing the offending drug (either drugs of abuse or medications) or the appropriate replacement and taper of a cross-reacting drug to minimize a withdrawal syndrome. Delirium in the elderly is frequently multifactorial and requires correction of a multitude of medical conditions.

In addition to addressing the cause of a delirium, oral, intramuscular, or intravenous haloperidol is of great use in treating agitation. Low doses of short-acting benzodiazepines can be used sparingly. Providing the

---

TABLE 8-3
Delirium Versus Dementia

	Delirium	Dementia
Onset	Hours to days	Weeks to years
Course/duration	Fluctuates within a day. May last hours to weeks*	Stable within a day. May be permanent, reversible or progressive over weeks to years
Attention	Impaired	May be impaired
Cognition	Impaired memory, orientation, language	Impaired memory, orientation, language, executive function
Perception	Hallucination, illusions, misinterpretations	Hallucinations, delusions
Sleep/wake	Disturbed, may have complete day/night reversal	Disturbed, may have no pattern
Mood/emotion	Labile affect	Labile affect; mood disturbances
Sundowning	Frequent	Frequent
Identified precipitant	Likely precipitant is present	Identifiable precipitant not required

*DSM-IV does not specify a limit for the duration for delirium; clinical experience suggests resolution within days to weeks, in most cases.

patient with a brightly lighted room with orienting cues such as names, clocks, and calendars is also useful.

Key Points

Delirium

1. Is a disorder of attention and cognition;
2. Has an abrupt onset and a variable course;
3. Has an identifiable precipitant;
4. Predicts a greater than 40% 1-year mortality rate.

▶ DEMENTIA

Dementia is characterized by the presence of **memory impairment** in the presence of other **cognitive defects.** Dementia is categorized according to its etiology (see Table 8-1). It can arise as a result of a specific disease entity, for example Alzheimer's disease or HIV infection; a general medical condition; a substance-related condition; or have multiple etiologies. The definitive cause may not be determined until autopsy.

Etiology

The etiology of dementia generally is brain neuronal loss that may be due to neuronal degeneration or to cell death secondary to trauma, infarction, hypoxia infection, or hydrocephalus. Table 8-1 lists the major discrete illnesses known to produce dementia. In addition, there are a large number of general medical, substance-related, and multifactorial causes of dementia.

▶ EPIDEMIOLOGY

The prevalence of dementia of all types is about 2% to 4% over age 65, increasing with age to a prevalence of about 20% over age 85. Specific epidemiologic factors relating to disease-specific causes of dementia are listed in Table 8-4.

Clinical Manifestations

History and Mental Status Examination

Dementia is diagnosed in the presence of multiple cognitive defects not better explained by another diagnosis. The presence of memory loss is required; in addition, one or more cognitive defects in the categories of aphasia, apraxia, agnosia, and disturbance in executive function must be present. Table 8-3 compares characteristics of dementia to those of delirium. Dementia often develops insidiously over the course of weeks to years (although it may be abrupt after head trauma or vascular insult). Individuals with dementia usually have a stable presentation over brief periods of

TABLE 8-4	
Specific Diseases Associated with Dementia	
Disease	Description
Alzheimer's	Most common cause of dementia, accounts for greater than 50% of all cases. Risk factors are familial, Down's syndrome, prior head trauma, increasing age. Pathology reveals cortical atrophy, neurofibrillary tangles, amyloid plaques, granulovacuolar degeneration , loss of basal forebrain cholinergic nuclei. Course is progressive, death occurs in 8–10 years after onset.
Vascular	Second most common cause of dementia. Risk factors are cardiovascular and cerebrovascular disease. Neuroimaging reveals multiple areas of neuronal damage. Neurological exam reveals focal findings. Course can be rapid onset or more slowly progressive. Deficits are not reversible, but progress can be halted with appropriate treatment of vascular disease.
HIV	Limited to those cases caused by direct action of HIV on the brain; associated illnesses, such as meningitis, lymphoma, toxoplasmosis producing dementia are categorized under dementia due to general medical conditions. Primarily affects white matter and cortex.
Head trauma	Most common among young males. Extent of dementia is determined by degree of brain damage. Deficits are stable unless there is repeated head trauma.
Parkinson's	Occurs in 20%–60% of individuals with Parkinson's disease. Bradyphrenia (slowed thinking) is common. Some individuals also have pathology at autopsy consistent with Alzheimer's dementia.
Huntington's	Risk factors are familial, autosomal dominant on chromosome 4. Onset commonly in mid 30s. Emotional lability is prominent. Caudate atrophy is present on autopsy.
Pick's	Onset at age 50–60. Frontal and temporal atrophy are prominent on neuroimaging.
Creutzfeldt-Jakob	Ten percent of cases are familial. Onset age 40–60. Prion is thought to be agent of transmission. Clinical triad of dementia, myoclonus, and abnormal EEG. Rapidly progressive. Spongiform encephalopathy is present at autopsy.

time, although they also may have nocturnal worsening of symptoms ("sundowning"). Memory impairment often is greatest for short-term memory. Recall of names frequently is impaired, as is recognition of familiar objects. Executive functions of organization and planning may be lost. Paranoia, hallucinations, and delusions often are present. Eventually, individuals with dementia may be comemute, incontinent, and bedridden.

Differential Diagnosis

Dementia should be differentiated from delirium. In addition, dementia should be differentiated from those developmental disorders (such as mental retardation) with impaired cognition. Individuals with major depression and psychosis can appear demented; they only warrant a diagnosis of dementia if their cognitive impairment cannot be fully attributed to the primary psychiatric illness.

A critical component of differential diagnosis in dementia is to distinguish pseudodementia associated with depression. Although there are many precise criteria for separating the two disorders, neuropsychological testing may be needed to make an accurate diagnosis. In pseudodementia, mood symptoms are prominent and patients may complain extensively of memory impairment. They characteristically give "I don't know" answers to mental status examination queries but may answer correctly if pressed. Memory is intact with rehearsal in pseudodementia, but not so in dementia.

Management

Dementia from reversible, or treatable, causes should be managed first by treating the underlying cause of the dementia; rehabilitation may be required for residual deficits. Reversible (or partially reversible) causes of dementia include normal pressure hydrocephalus; neurosyphilis; HIV infection; and thiamine, folate, vitamin B_{12}, and niacin deficiency. Vascular dementias may not be reversible, but their progress can be halted in some cases. Nonreversible dementias usually are managed by placing the patient in a safe environment and by medications targeted at associated symptoms. Tacrine, ananticholinesterase inhibitor, has some efficacy in treating memory loss in dementia of the Alzheimer's type. High-potency antipsychotics (in low doses) are used when agitation, paranoia, and hallucinations are present. Low-dose benzodiazepines and trazodone are often used for anxiety, agitation, or insomnia.

Key Points

Dementia

1. Is a disorder of memory impairment coupled to other cognitive defects;
2. Has a gradual onset and progressive course;
3. May be caused by a variety of illnesses;
4. Predisposes to delirium.

▶ AMNESTIC DISORDERS

Amnestic disorder is an isolated disturbance of memory without impairment of other cognitive functions. It may be due to a general medical condition or substance related.

Etiology

Amnestic disorders are caused by **general medical conditions** or **substance use**. Common general medical conditions include head trauma, hypoxia, herpes simplex encephalitis, and posterior cerebral artery infarction. Amnestic disorders often are associated with damage of the mammillary bodies, fornix, and hippocampus. Bilateral damage to these structures produces the most severe deficits. Amnestic disorders due to substance-related causes may be due to substance abuse, prescribed or over the counter medications, or accidental exposure to toxins. Alcohol abuse is a leading cause of substance-related amnestic disorder. Persistent alcohol use may lead to thiamine deficiency and induce a Wernicke-Korsakoff syndrome. If properly treated, the acute symptoms of ataxia, abnormal eye movements, and confusion may resolve, leaving a residual amnestic disorder called Korsakoff's psychosis (alcohol-induced persistent amnestic disorder).

Epidemiology

Individuals affected by a general medical condition or alcoholism are at risk for amnestic disorders.

Clinical Manifestations

History and Mental Status Examination

Amnestic disorders present as **deficits in memory**, either in the inability to recall previously learned information or the inability to retain new information. The cognitive defect must be limited to memory alone; if additional cognitive defects are present, a diagnosis of dementia or delirium should be considered. In addition to defect in memory, there must be an **identifiable cause** for the amnestic disorder (i.e., the presence of a general medical condition or substance use likely to be causative of the amnestic disorder).

Differential Diagnosis

Delirium and dementia are the major differential diagnostic considerations.

Management

The general medical condition is treated whenever possible to prevent further neurologic damage; in the case of a substance-related amnestic disorder, avoiding re-exposure to the substance responsible for the amnestic disorder is critical. Pharmacotherapy may be directed at treating associated anxiety or mood difficulties. Patients should be placed in a safe structured environment with frequent memory cues.

Key Points

Amnestic disorders

1. Are disorders in memory alone;
2. Are caused by identifiable precipitants;
3. Are reversible in some cases.

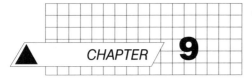

CHAPTER 9

Miscellaneous Disorders

*M*iscellaneous disorders does not refer to any official *Diagnostic and Statistical Manual of Mental Disorders*, 4th edition (DSM-IV) classification but rather refers to psychiatric diagnoses not covered elsewhere in this book. Generally, these diagnoses are either less common, less understood, or less frequently the focus of psychiatric practice than the disorders previously covered. Although many of these disorders are not uncommon, they may only come to psychiatric attention for a variety of reasons (e.g., they may be treated by other medical specialists, patients may not mention them, or they may not be detected adequately). Table 9-1 lists the categories of disorders discussed in this chapter.

▶ DISSOCIATIVE DISORDERS

Dissociative disorders are characterized by disturbances in the integration of mental functions. These disturbances are manifest by loss of memory for personal information or identity, division of consciousness and personality into separate parts, and altered perception of the environment or one's sense of reality. Table 9-2 lists and defines the dissociative disorders.

Dissociative Amnesia

In dissociative amnesia, an individual develops a temporary inability to recall important personal information. The amnesia is more extensive than forgetfulness and is not caused by another medical or psychiatric condition (e.g., head trauma). The inability to recall information may take several forms. In **localized** amnesia, information is lost for a specific time period (e.g., a time associated with trauma). In **selective** amnesia, some information during a given time period is retained but other information is lost. In **generalized**

TABLE 9-1	
Miscellaneous Disorders	
Dissociative disorders	
Somatoform disorders	
Adjustment disorders	
Sexual and gender identity disorders	
Sleep disorders	
Factitious disorders/malingering	

TABLE 9-2	
Dissociative Disorders	
Dissociative amnesia	Temporary inability to recall important personal information; more serious than simple forgetfulness.
Dissociative fugue	Amnesia for one's identity coupled with sudden unexplained travel away from home.
Dissociative identity disorder	Presence of two or more separate personalities that recurrently take control of a person's behavior.
Depersonalization disorder	Pervasive sense of being detached from or being outside of one's body.

amnesia, personal information is lost for the entire life span. In **continuous** amnesia, there is an inability to recall information from a single point in time to the present. In **systematized** amnesia, particular categories of information are lost to retrieval.

Dissociative amnesia is more common in people exposed to trauma, for example, exposure to battle or natural disaster.

Dissociative Fugue

Dissociative fugue is an amnestic disorder characterized by sudden unexplained travel away from one's home, coupled with amnesia for one's identity. In this condition, patients do not appear mentally ill or otherwise impaired in any other mental function, including memory. In fact, patients are quite capable of negotiating the complexities of travel and interaction with others. In rare cases, individuals will establish a completely new identity in their new home. Dissociative fugue is typically precipitated by a severe trauma or stressor and eventually remits without treatment.

Dissociative Identity Disorder

Dissociative identity disorder (formerly called multiple personality disorder) is a controversial diagnostic entity in psychiatry. The diagnosis of dissociative identity disorder requires the presence of two or more separate personalities (alters) that recurrently take control of an individual's behavior. Individuals with this disorder often will have amnesia for important personal information (also known as "losing time"). The various personalities (the average number by available surveys is seven distinct personalities) may be unaware of the existence of one another and thus may be quite confused as to how they arrived at certain places or why they cannot recall personal events. At other times, one or more personalities may be aware of the others, a condition known as coconsciousness. Some personalities may display conversion symptoms or self-mutilating behavior. The alters may be of varying ages and different gender and demeanor.

Dissociative identity disorder is most common in females and has a chronic course. Individuals with dissociative identity disorder are highly suggestible and easily hypnotized. Most report a childhood history of severe physical or sexual abuse. Satanic or cult abuse reports also are not uncommon. In many cases, these reports of abuse cannot be verified, leading many clinicians to believe that individuals with dissociative identity disorder may suffer from memories of events that did not occur. Whether these memories are true or false, they cause a great deal of suffering.

Disagreement over the very nature of dissociative identify disorder has led to diverging treatment opinions. Some clinicians believe that ignoring the different personalities will cause them to recede, based on the notion that the easy suggestibility of these patients will lead to reinforcement of alters if they are discussed. Others believe that long-term psychotherapy, exploring the various personalities, and integrating them into a whole person is the treatment of choice.

Depersonalization Disorder

Depersonalization disorder is characterized by "persistent or recurrent experiences of feeling detached from and as if one is an outside observer of one's mental processes or body" (DSM-IV). Individuals with this disorder may complain of a sense of detachment, of feeling mechanical or automated, and of absence of affect or sensation. Individuals with depersonalization disorder are easily hypnotized and prone to dissociate.

▶ SOMATOFORM DISORDERS

Somatoform disorders are characterized by the presence of physical signs or symptoms but without medical cause. In addition, they are *not* willfully produced by the individual. The somatoform disorders are listed and defined in Table 9-3.

Somatization Disorder

Somatization disorder is diagnosed when an individual has multiple medical complaints that are not the result of medical illness. The specific DSM-IV criteria are narrow and specific, requiring

▲ Pain in four different body sites or involving four different body functions;

▲ Two gastrointestinal symptoms (other than pain);

▲ One sexual symptom (other than pain);

▲ One pseudoneurologic symptom (other than pain).

In addition, some symptoms must have begun before age 30 and persist for several years. Individuals with somatization disorder often have a history of complex medical and surgical treatments that actually may lead to iatrogenic complications of treatment. Patients with somatoform disorder frequently have multiple physicians, are high users of office and hospital visits, and may seek disability because of their conviction that they are severely and chronically medically ill.

This disorder is more common in females (approximately 80% of cases), and its incidence is increased in first-degree relatives of those with somatization disorder. Familial and genetic studies also have shown that

TABLE 9-3	
Somatoform Disorders	
Somatization disorder	Chronic multiple medical complaints that include pain, gastrointestinal disturbance, sexual symptoms, and pseudoneurologic symptoms that are not due to a medical illness.
Undifferentiated somatoform disorder	A less severe form of somatization disorder; involves fewer complaints and briefer course.
Conversion disorder	Complaints involving sensory (such as numbness) and voluntary motor (such as paralysis) function that are not due to neurologic dysfunction.
Pain disorder	Pain is the major complaint. If medical causes are present, psychological factors have a major role in mediating the expression and impact of pain.
Hypochondriasis	Preoccupation with having a serious disease based on a misinterpretation of bodily function and sensation.
Body dysmorphic disorder	Excessive concern with a perceived defect in appearance.

Sexual and Gender Identity Disorders

Sexual Dysfunctions	Paraphilias
Sexual desire disorders	Exhibitionism
Hypoactive sexual desire	Fetishism
disorder	Frotteurism
Sexual aversion disorder	Pedophilia
Sexual arousal disorders	Sexual masochism
Female sexual arousal	Sexual sadism
disorder	Transvestic fetishism
Male sexual arousal	Voyeurism
disorder	
Orgasmic disorders	
Female orgasmic disorder	
Male orgasmic disorder	
Premature ejaculation	
Sexual pain disorders	
Dyspareunia	
Vaginismus	
Sexual dysfunction due to a	
general medical condition	
Substance-induced sexual	
dysfunction	

TABLE 9-5

Sexual Response Cycle

Desire	Initial stage of sexual response; consists of sexual fantasies and the urge to have sex.
Excitement	Consists of physiologic arousal and feeling of sexual pleasure.
Orgasm	Peaking sexual pleasure; usually associated with ejaculation in males.
Resolution	Physiologic relaxation associated with sense of well-being. In males, there is usually a refractory period for further excitement and orgasm.

TABLE 9-6

Specific Sexual Dysfunctions

Sexual desire disorders	
Hypoactive sexual desire disorder	Sexual fantasy and desire for sex are very low or absent.
Sexual aversion disorder	Aversion to genital sexual contact with another person.
Sexual arousal disorders	
Female sexual arousal disorder	Inadequate vaginal lubrication and inadequate engorgement of external genitalia.
Male erectile disorder	Inability to attain or maintain an erection.
Orgasmic disorders	
Female orgasmic disorder	Orgasm is absent or delayed. Sexual excitement phase is normal.
Male orgasmic disorder	Orgasm is absent or delayed. Sexual excitement phase is normal.
Premature ejaculation	Orgasm and ejaculation occur early and with minimal stimulation.
Sexual pain disorders	
Dyspareunia	Genital pain in association with sexual intercourse.
Vaginismus	Involuntary contraction of external vaginal musculature as a result of attempted penetration.

male relatives of individuals with somatization disorder have an increased incidence of antisocial personality disorder and substance abuse. Adoption studies suggest genetic influences in this disorder.

Various theories have been proposed to explain this disorder. Early psychoanalytic work focused on repressed instincts as causative; more modern theorists propose that somatization symptoms may represent a means of nonverbal interpersonal communication. Biologic findings have revealed abnormal cortical function in some individuals with this disorder.

▶ ADJUSTMENT DISORDERS

Adjustment disorders are symptoms (changes in emotional state or behaviors) that arise in response to an identified psychosocial stressor. Adjustment disorder is not diagnosed if the symptoms occurred in response to a psychosocial stressor so severe that an individual meets criteria for another axis I disorder (e.g., major depression). Symptoms in response to bereavement do not meet criteria for the diagnosis of adjustment disorder. Adjustment disorders occur within 3 months of the identified stressor and usually resolve within 6 months, unless the stressor(s) become chronic.

▶ SEXUAL AND GENDER IDENTITY DISORDERS

These disorders are divided into sexual dysfunctions, paraphilia, and gender identity disorders. Sexual dys-

functions and paraphilia are further classified as outlined in Table 9-4.

Sexual Dysfunctions

Sexual dysfunctions are those sexual disorders associated with alterations in the sexual response cycle or with pain associated with sexual activity (Table 9-5). The specific sexual dysfunctions are defined in Table 9-6.

Paraphilias

Paraphilia (Table 9-7) include sexual disorders related to culturally unusual sexual activity. A key criterion for the diagnosis of a paraphilia (as in all psychiatric disorders) is that an individual must **experience significant distress or impairment in social or occupational functioning.** In other words, an individual with unusual sexual practices who does not suffer significant distress or impairment would not be diagnosed with a psychiatric illness.

Gender Identity Disorders

Gender identity disorder remains a controversial diagnosis in psychiatry. Individuals with this disorder experience distress and interpersonal impairment as a result of their desire to be a member of the opposite sex. Criterion for the diagnosis require a pervasive cross-gender identification and persistent discomfort with one's assigned sex. In addition, the diagnosis is made only in those individuals who do not have an intersex condition (e.g., ambiguous genitalia). Children with this disorder may engage in gender atypical play; adults may assume the societal role, dress, and behavior associated with the opposite sex. In addition, patients with gender identity disorder may seek sex reassignment surgery and hormonal supplements. Individuals with gender identity disorder appear to have the same range of sexual orientations as do persons without this disorder.

▶ SLEEP DISORDERS

Sleep disorders are illnesses related to alterations in the sleep wake cycle (Table 9-9) and often have effects on mood, cognitive, somatic, and general performance. Table 9-8 outlines the classification of sleep disorders. Sleep disorders are categorized into primary and secondary sleep disorders. Primary sleep disorders are those disorders occurring as a direct result of disturbances in the sleep-wake cycle. They are divided into two categories: dyssomnias and parasomnias. Secondary sleep disorders are a consequence of other mental disorders (e.g., depression) due to general medical conditions (e.g., somatic pain) or substance use (e.g., caffeine).

Dyssomnias

Dyssomnias are five primary sleep disorders consisting of disturbances in initiating and maintaining sleep, feeling rested or refreshed after sleep, or sleeping excessively. Table 9-10 defines the key characteristics of each disorder.

TABLE 9-7

Paraphilias

Exhibitionism	Sexual excitement is derived from exposing one's genitals to a stranger.
Fetishism	Nonliving objects are the focus of intense sexual arousal in fantasy or behavior.
Frotteurism	Sexual excitement is derived by rubbing one's genitals against or by sexually touching a nonconsenting stranger.
Pedophilia	Sexual excitement is derived from fantasy or behavior involving sex with prepubescent children.
Sexual masochism	Sexual excitement is derived from fantasy or behavior involving being the recipient of humiliation, bondage, or pain.
Sexual sadism	Sexual excitement is derived from fantasy or behavior involving inflicting suffering/humiliation on another.
Transvestic fetishism	Sexual excitement (in heterosexual males) is derived from fantasy or behavior involving wearing women's clothing.
Voyeurism	Sexual excitement is derived from fantasy or behavior involving the observation of unsuspecting individuals undressing, naked, or having sex.

TABLE 9-8

Sleep Disorders

Primary Sleep Disorders	Secondary Sleep Disorders
Dyssomnias	Sleep disorder related to
Primary insomnia	another mental disorder
Primary hypersomnia	Sleep disorder due to a
Narcolepsy	general medical condition
Breathing-related sleep	Substance-induced sleep
disorder	disorder
Circadian rhythm sleep	
disorder	
Parasomnias	
Nightmare disorder	
Sleep terror disorder	
Sleepwalking disorder	

Parasomnias

Parasomnias are a triad of sleep disorders associated with complex behavioral events either occurring during sleep or that arouse one from sleep. The disorders are defined in Table 9-10.

▶ FACTITIOUS DISORDERS

A factitious disorder is one in which an individual willfully produces signs or symptoms of a medical or psychiatric illness to assume the sick role and its associated gratifications. This should be differentiated from conversion disorder (which is not willful) and **malingering**, which is simply lying about signs or symptoms to obtain gain different from that of the sick role (e.g., to avoid the military or for monetary gain).

TABLE 9-9
Sleep Stages

Nonrapid eye movement

Stage 0	Awake. *α dominates,*	
ℬ Stage 1	Very light* sleep, transition from wakefulness to sleep. Drowsy.	
Stage 2 *Sleep Spindles @*	Medium depth of sleep, occupies about half the night in adults. Serves as a transition stage between rapid eye movement (REM) and delta sleep.	
Delta	Slow wave sleep, composed of stages 3 and 4.	
Stage 3	Consists of a moderate amount of delta wave activity; deeper sleep than stage 2.	
Stage 4	Increased delta wave activity over stage 3. Very deep stage of sleep.	
REM	Dream sleep. EEG is active, mimicking that of the waking stage. Depth of sleep is greater than stage 2 but probably less than delta.	

*Depth of sleep as used here is not a precise term but generally refers to ease of arousability (i.e., how hard would it be to awaken an individual from a particular stage). However, the ease of arousability is in part due to the type of stimulus used (e.g., noise versus touch).

TABLE 9-10
Primary Sleep Disorders

Dyssomnias

Primary insomnia	Difficulty falling asleep, staying asleep, or sleeping but feeling as if one has not rested during sleep.
Primary hypersomnia	Excess sleepiness, either sleeping too long at one setting or persistent daytime sleepiness not relieved by napping.
Narcolepsy	Sleep attacks during the daytime coupled to REM sleep intrusions or cataplexy (sudden, reversible bilateral loss of skeletal muscle tone). Daytime naps relieve sleepiness.
Breathing-related sleep disorder	Abnormal breathing during sleep leads to sleep disruption and daytime sleepiness.
Circadian rhythm sleep disorder	Sleep disturbance due to a mismatch between a person's intrinsic circadian rhythm and external sleep wake demands.
Parasomnias	
Nightmare disorder	Repeated episodes of scary dreams that wake one from sleep, usually occur during *REM* sleep.
Sleep terror disorder	Repeated episodes of apparent terror during sleep; an individual may sit up, scream, or cry out and appear extremely frightened. They do not usually awaken during the attack. Occurs during *delta* sleep.
Sleepwalking disorder	Recurrent sleepwalking, often coupled to other complex motor activity.

CHAPTER 10

Special Clinical Situations

▶ SUICIDE ATTEMPTS

Epidemiology

Suicide is the eighth leading cause of death in the United States. Approximately 75 people commit suicide each day in the United States (25,000 per year). Many more people attempt suicide. The overall suicide rate has remained stable in the United States over the past 15 years. The risk of suicide peaks in the third decade of life. Although the rate of suicide in teenagers aged 15 to 19 is low compared with the general adult population, the rate of teen suicide has risen dramatically in the last 40 years (from 2.7 per 100,000 in 1950 to 11.3 per 100,000 in 1988).

Risk Factors

Studies have demonstrated that the overwhelming majority of people who commit suicide have a mental illness (most often a mood disorder or chronic alcoholism). The first-degree relatives of people who have committed suicide are at a much higher risk of committing suicide themselves. Suicide risk increases with age. In men, suicides peak after age 45; in women, most suicides occur after age 55. The elderly account for 25% of the suicides, although they represent only 10% of the population. Overall, men are more successful at completing suicide, perhaps related to their more lethal methods (shooting, hanging, jumping); women often overdose or attempt drowning. Married persons have a lower risk of suicide than singles. Suicide is more common among higher social classes, whites, and certain professional groups (physicians, dentists, musicians, law enforcement officers, lawyers, and insurance agents). Biologic risk factors include low levels of 5-hydroxyindoleacetic acid in the cerebrospinal fluid of patients who have committed suicide by violent means. Among psychological risk factors, hopelessness has been shown to be one of the most reliable indicators of long-term suicide risk.

Clinical Manifestations

History and Mental Status Examination

Most often, a suicide attempt is self-evident at presentation, either because the patient or family indicate that such an event has occurred or because there is an acute medical or surgical emergency (i.e., overdose or wrist laceration). Always obtain further details from the patient and any witnesses to provide a full history of the antecedents and the act itself. Occasionally, a patient will present to a physician in a more subtle way, with nonspecific complaints. Careful inquiry may reveal that the patient has taken an overdose of a medication with delayed lethality (such as acetaminophen).

Patients who have attempted suicide deserve thorough psychiatric evaluation. Psychiatric history and mental status examination should inquire explicitly for depressive symptoms, such as suicidal thoughts, intent, and plans. The details of the suicide attempt are critical to understanding the risk of a future suicide. Patients who carefully plan the attempt, use particularly violent means, and isolate themselves so as not to be found alive are at particularly high risk of future suicide completion.

Differential Diagnosis

Patients who attempt suicide most commonly suffer from depression, schizophrenia, alcoholism, or personality disorders (or comorbidities of the above). However, patients who do not meet criteria for any of these disorders can and do attempt or commit suicide, especially if they have any of the risk factors (e.g., hopelessness).

Management

Suicidal ideation always should be taken seriously. Suicidal patients often are fraught with ambivalence over whether to live or die, and intervention and effective treatment can be life-saving. Most actively suicidal patients require hospitalization on a locked unit for their safety. Potentially lethal items should be held securely by nursing staff, and the patient should be observed carefully for the risk of elopement. Treatment of the underlying disorder or distress derives from accurate diagnosis (antidepressants or electroconvulsive therapy [ECT] for depression; antipsychotics and/or mood stabilizers for bipolar disorder, psychotic depression, or schizophrenia).

Patients at lower risk of suicide often can be managed as outpatients if close follow-up is available, family members are supportive, and a treatment alliance exists. Frequent meetings with treaters, eliminating the means of suicide (firearms, potentially toxic prescription pills), and enlisting spouses or other family members are essential elements of outpatient treatment.

▶ SPOUSAL ABUSE

Abuse between spouses or partners can take several forms: physical, sexual, and emotional. Physical abuse or battering most often is perpetrated by a male on a female partner, but women do batter men and abuse occurs in homosexual relationships.

Epidemiology

Spousal abuse is estimated to occur in 2 to 12 million U.S. households. Some studies estimate that nearly one-third of all women have been beaten by their husband at least once during their marriage. Many battered women eventually are murdered by their spouses or boyfriends.

Risk Factors

There is a strong association between alcohol abuse and domestic violence. More than 50% of abusers, and many of the abused, have a history of alcohol or other drug abuse. As children, most abusers lived in violent homes where either they witnessed or were themselves battered. The victims of abuse, more often than not, also are products of violent homes. Pregnant women are at elevated risk for spousal abuse, often directed at their abdomens.

Clinical Manifestations

History and Physical and Mental Status Examination

Many victims of abuse are reluctant to report abusive episodes because they fear retaliation, believe they are deserving of abuse, or do not believe that help will be effective. Victims of abuse also often are mistreated in ways that prevent them from escaping the abusive relationship. They are intimidated, maligned, coerced, and isolated by the abuser. Leaving an abusive relationship is thwarted by financial concerns, the welfare of children, fear of being alone, or the threat of further battering.

Patients may present in the company of their abuser for the treatment of "accidental" lacerations, contusions, fractures, or more severe trauma. Unless the patient is asked tactfully in the absence of the abuser, she or he is unlikely to reveal the true cause of injuries.

Physical examination should include examination of the skin for contusions (especially of the face and breasts) and a genital examination. The mental status examination should be alert to the appropriateness of the patient's and spouse's reactions to the "accident."

Management

The goal of treatment is to end the violence (i.e., both partners must agree to treatment) or enable the woman to leave the relationship. Either option is difficult to achieve. Social agencies must be enlisted to aid in child protection and custody if the latter option is chosen.

Patients who refuse help should be told what emergency services are available and how they may be accessed. Unfortunately, women are most at risk for serious injury or homicide when they attempt to leave the abusive relationship.

▶ ELDER ABUSE

Approximately 10% of those older than 65 are abused. Victims usually live with their assailants, who often are their children. Mistreatment includes abuse and neglect and takes physical, psychological, financial, and material forms. The abuser may withhold food, clothing, or other necessities or beat, sexually molest, or emotional abuse the victim.

As with spousal abuse, the elder person often is reluctant to reveal the abuse. Clinicians should be alert to the signs of abuse. Treatment involves appropriate medical and psychiatric services and social and legal services. Some states mandate reporting of elder abuse.

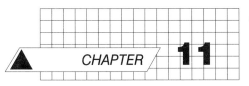

CHAPTER 11

Antipsychotics

$\pmb{A}$ntipsychotic medications are used commonly in medical and psychiatric practice. As a class, antipsychotics have in common their blockade of dopamine receptors and their potential for serious side effects if used inappropriately or without careful monitoring. The most commonly prescribed typical and atypical antipsychotics are listed in Table 11-1. Their relative potency, relative side-effect profile, and major adverse reactions also are described. **Typical** antipsychotics (also called neuroleptics for their tendency to cause movement disorders) generally are equally effective, although they differ in side-effect profiles and potency. **Atypical** antipsychotics (e.g., risperidone and clozapine) have fewer extrapyramidal side effects at therapeutic doses when compared with typical antipsychotics. Clozapine (and perhaps risperidone) is more effective than typical antipsychotics for the treatment of refractory psychotic disorders.

▶ INDICATIONS

Antipsychotics generally are effective in treating **positive** psychotic symptoms (e.g., hallucinations, bizarre behavior, delusions) **regardless of diagnostic category** (Table 11-2). For example, hallucinations in schizophrenia, in Alzheimer's disease, or secondary to cerebral toxicity or injury all respond to antipsychotic medications. Antipsychotics are thought to be less effective (with the exception of clozapine and possibly risperidone) in treating **negative** psychotic symptoms (e.g., amotivation, akinesia, affective blunting, social withdrawal). In addition to their role in treating psychotic symptoms, antipsychotics are used to treat some forms of nonpsychotic behavioral dyscontrol (e.g., organic brain syndromes, Alzheimer's, mental retardation), delirium, Gilles de la Tourette syndrome, and with transient psychotic symptoms as they appear in personality disorder patients.

TABLE 11-1
Commonly Prescribed Antipsychotics

Drug	Potency*	Histamine Sedative	α₁ Block Hypotensive	M₁ Block Anticholinergic	D₂ Block EPS	Other Adverse Reactions
Typical antipsychotics (dopamine antagonists)						
Thioridazine (Mellaril)	100	High	High	High	Low	Pigmentary retinopathy
Chlorpromazine (Thorazine)	100	High	High	Med	Low	
Perphenazine (Trilafon)	10	Low	Low	Low	Med	
Trifluoperazine (Stelazine)	5	Med	Low	Low	High	
Thiothixene (Navane)	5	Low	Low	Low	High	*good in Epilepsy*
Haloperidol (Haldol)	2	Low	Low	Low	High	*Avail. in Depot.*
Fluphenazine (Prolixin)	2	Med	Low	Low	High	
Atypical antipsychotics (serotonin/dopamine antagonists)						
D₄/5HT Clozapine (Clozaril)	100	High	High	High	Very low	Agranulocytosis
D₂/5HT Risperidone (Risperdal)	1	Low	Med	Low	Low	

*Potency is indicated as relative milligram dose equivalents (i.e., 100 mg of thioridazine is equivalent to 2 mg of haloperidol) and should not be confused with efficacy. All typical antipsychotics are thought to be equally efficacious. Efficacy for clozapine and risperidone is at least equal to and may be superior to typical antipsychotics.

Reproduced by permission from Hyman SE, Arana GW, Rosenbaum JF, Handbook of psychiatric drug therapy, 3rd ed. Antipsychotic drugs. Boston: Little, Brown and Company, 1991:8.

TABLE 11-2

Common Indications for Antipsychotic Usage

Psychotic disorders
  Schizophrenia
  Schizophreniform disorder
  Schizoaffective disorder
  Delusional disorder
  Brief psychotic disorders
Mood disorders
  Depression with psychotic symptoms
  Mania with psychosis
  Treatment resistant mania
  Substance-induced mood disorder with psychosis
Personality disorders
  For transient psychotic symptoms   *schizotypal.*
Other disorders
  Organic brain syndromes
  Dementia
  Gilles de la Tourette syndrome

Reproduced by permission from Hyman SE, Arana GW, Rosenbaum JF, Handbook of psychiatric drug therapy, 3rd ed. Antipsychotic drugs. Boston: Little, Brown and Company, 1991:15.

Mechanism of Action

The most prominent theory on the mechanism of action of antipsychotics is **the dopamine hypothesis of schizophrenia**. This hypothesis purports that dopaminergic hyperactivity leads to psychosis. Evidence supporting a role for hyperdopaminergic states in schizophrenia (and presumably other psychotic states) is as follows: antipsychotic potency of traditional antipsychotics correlates highly with their potency of dopamine receptor blockade, individuals with schizophrenia have an increased number of brain dopamine receptors, and dopamine agonist drugs (e.g., amphetamine) can induce or exacerbate existing psychosis.

The mechanism of action of antipsychotics is often much broader than simple dopamine blockade, which accounts for the numerous side effects and the finding that their action in the brain is not well correlated with regions thought to give rise to psychotic symptoms. In addition, newer drugs such as clozapine and risperidone have prominent serotonin (5-hydroxy-tryptamine-2 [$5HT_2$]) receptor blockade. It is unclear whether this serotonin blockade imparts antipsychotic efficacy or simply helps prevent extrapyramidal side effects.

Typical Antipsychotics (Dopamine Antagonists)

The antipsychotic potency of **typical** antipsychotics (and risperidone) correlates with their affinity for the D_2 receptor. Figure 11-1 is a schematic diagram of the proposed brain pathways affected by **typical** antipsychotics. Dopamine-containing axons arising from brain stem nuclei (the ventral tegmental area and substantia nigra) project to the basal ganglia, frontal cortex, and limbic areas. Typical antipsychotics block D_2 receptors (as does risperidone). Blockade of dopamine in the cortical and limbic areas results in reduction in psychotic symptoms, whereas blockade of dopamine in the basal ganglia produces extrapyramidal side effects. Although antipsychotics, especially lower potency medications, may have an initial sedative effect, their antipsychotic action is not immediate and takes several days to several weeks to peak.

Atypical Antipsychotics (Serotonin/Dopamine Antagonists)

At present, in the United States two atypical antipsychotics are marketed; others are likely to be available soon. Antipsychotics are classified as atypical when they produce fewer movement side effects than typical antipsychotics. In addition to dopamine receptor blockade, atypical antipsychotics block serotonin receptors of the $5HT_2$ subtype. Figure 11-2 depicts the similarities and differences of the serotonin and

Figure 11-1 Pathways affected by typical antipsychotics.

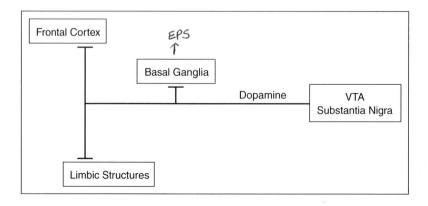

dopamine systems. Serotonin receptor blockade conveys some protection against extrapyramidal side effects and may impart antipsychotic efficacy. Risperidone is similar to typical neuroleptics in that it is a very potent blocker of the D_2 receptor. Clozapine, conversely, is a potent blocker of the D_4 receptor and has less D_2 affinity. The D_4 receptor blockade may confer upon clozapine its broader therapeutic qualities.

Choice of Medication

Because all antipsychotics are considered efficacious, medication choice should be based on prior patient or family member response, side effect profile (patient tolerance), and available form (i.e., elixiror IM or IM depot availability). At present, clozapine is the only medication clearly shown to be superior in patients who have failed typical antipsychotics. Fluphenazine and haloperidol are available in depot preparations, which are given intramuscularly every 2 to 4 weeks.

Therapeutic Monitoring

Patients on antipsychotics should be monitored closely for adverse drug reactions. Particularly important are neurologic side effects such as akathisia (restlessness), neuroleptic malignant syndrome (NMS), and extrapyramidal symptoms (EPS). Patients taking antipsychotics that lower seizure threshold should be carefully monitored for seizure activity. Individuals taking clozapine must have weekly white blood cell counts to monitor for the development of a granulocytosis. Clozapine must be discontinued immediately in patients demonstrating this potentially fatal reaction.

Blood levels generally have been of little use in monitoring antipsychotic efficacy, in part because some medications have many active metabolites. Haloperidol levels have some utility in patients who have side effects at low doses or who fail to respond to high doses. Noncompliance often is the cause of apparent therapeutic failure. Clozapine levels also are frequently used.

The duration of therapy depends on the nature and the severity of the patient's illness. Many disorders, such as schizophrenia, require maintenance antipsychotic therapy. Because of the serious sequela associated with long-term antipsychotic use, maintenance therapy should be used only after a careful risk-to-benefit analysis with the patient and involved family.

Side Effects and Adverse Drug Reactions

Side effects of antipsychotics are a major consideration in physician prescribing. Patients who cannot bear the side effects of medications are noncompliant and suffer greater rates of relapse and recurrence. Certain side effects such a ssedation can be useful to a patient with insomnia or severe agitation but also can limit functioning. A comparison of side-effect profiles for commonly used antipsychotics is provided in Table 11-1. Descriptions of common side effects are described below. Further discussion of neurologic side effects is found in Chapter 16.

Anticholinergic Side Effects

Low-potency antipsychotics have the greatest anticholinergic side effects such as dry mouth, constipation, urinary retention, and blurred vision. The anticholinergic properties, however, counter the EPS. In some cases, anticholinergic delirium may occur, especially in the elderly, those with organic brain syndromes, or patients on other anticholinergic agents.

Reduced Seizure Threshold

Low-potency typical antipsychotics and clozapine are associated with lowering seizure threshold. Seizures

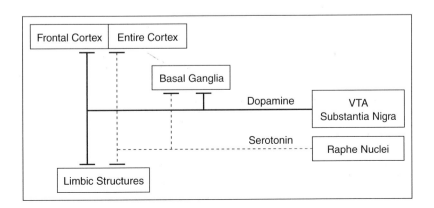

Figure 11-2 Pathways affected by atypical antipsychotics.

resulting from antipsychotic therapy are treated by changing medications, lowering the dose, or adding an antiseizure medication.

Hypotension

Orthostatic hypotension is particularly common with low-potency agents and risperidone. The hypotensive effect of antipsychotics generally is due to alpha-receptor blockade.

Agranulocytosis

Agranulocytosis has been associated most commonly with clozapine. Because of the potentially fatal nature of this adverse effect, clozapine distribution is regulated and requires a weekly complete blood count with differential to monitor for neutropenia.

Cardiac Side Effects

Low-potency antipsychotics and risperidone may cause QT prolongation (with risk of torsades de pointes). Nonspecific electrocardiographic changes also may occur.

Movement Disorders

Movement disorders such as dystonia, EPS, akathisia, NMS, and tardive dyskinesia may occur and are discussed further in Chapter 16.

Other Side Effects

Skin and ocular pigmentation are common side effects of neuroleptics, as is increased photosensitivity. Thioridazine can cause pigmentary retinopathy at high doses. Increased **prolactin** levels (and sequela) may also occur.

Key Points

Antipsychotics

1. Are used to treat the psychotic symptoms found in a wide range of disorders;

2. Are equally effective but differ in potency (with the exception of clozapine and possibly risperidone);

3. Have the potential for serious side effects.

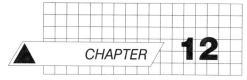

CHAPTER 12

Antidepressants

Antidepressants are used commonly in medical and psychiatric practice. As a class, antidepressants have in common their ability to treat major depressive illness. Most antidepressants also treat <u>panic</u> disorder and other <u>anxiety</u> disorders. Some antidepressants effectively treat <u>obsessive-compulsive disorder</u> and a variety of other conditions (see indications below).

The most commonly prescribed antidepressants are listed in Table 12-1. Antidepressants are subdivided into groups: selective serotonin reuptake inhibitors (SSRIs), tricyclic antidepressants (TCAs), monoamine oxidase inhibitors (MAOIs), and other antidepressant compounds with a variety of mechanisms of action. Antidepressants are typically thought to act on either the serotonin or norepinephrine systems or both. Choice of medications is typically dependent on diagnosis, history of response (in patient or relative), and the side-effect profile of the medication. Antidepressant effects typically are not seen until 2 to 4 weeks into treatment. Side effects must be carefully monitored, especially for TCAs and MAOIs.

▶ INDICATIONS

Table 12-2 lists the indications for antidepressants. The main indication for antidepressant medications is the *Diagnostic and Statistical Manual of Mental Disorders*, 4th edition (DSM-IV) defined major depressive disorder. Antidepressants are used in the treatment of all subtypes of depression, including depressed phase of bipolar disorder, psychotic depression (in combination with an antipsychotic medication), and atypical depression (see Chapter 2). Antidepressants also are indicated for the prevention of recurrent depressive episodes.

Antidepressant medications may be effective in the treatment of patients with dysthymic disorder, especially when there are clear neurovegetative signs or a history of response to antidepressants.

TABLE 12-1

Commonly Prescribed Antidepressants

Drug (Brand Name)	Starting Dosage*	Maximum Dosage*
SSRIs		
Fluoxetine (Prozac)	5–20 mg/day	80 mg/day
Sertraline (Zoloft)	25–50 mg/day	200 mg/day
Paroxetine (Paxil)	10–20 mg/day	50 mg/day
Fluvoxamine (Luvox)	25–50 mg qhs	300 mg qhs
TCAs		
Nortriptyline (Pamelor)	10–25 mg/day	150 mg/day
Imipramine (Tofranil)	10–50 mg/day	300 mg/day
Desipramine (Norpramin)	10–25 mg/day	300 mg/day
Clomipramine (Anafranil)	25–50 mg/day	250 mg/day
MAOIs		
Tranylcypromine (Parnate)	10–20 mg/day	60 mg/day
Phenelzine (Nardil)	15–30 mg/day	90 mg/day
Other antidepressants		
Bupropion (Wellbutrin)	75–100 mg/day	150 mg tid
Nefazodone (Serzone)	50–100 mg bid	600 mg/day
Venlafaxine (Effexor)	25 mg tid	125 mg tid

*Geriatric patients generally require lower doses.

Reproduced with permission from Stoll A, Psychopharmacology reference card I. 1996.

TABLE 12-2
Common Indications for Antidepressant Usage

Mood disorders
  Major depressive disorder
  Bipolar disorder, depressed phase
  Depression with psychotic symptoms
  Atypical depression
  Dysthymic disorder
  Mood disorder due to a general medical condition
Anxiety disorders
  Panic disorder with or without agoraphobia
  Obsessive-compulsive disorder   *Clomipramine*
Other disorders
  Bulimia   *SSRI*
  Neuropathic pain (tricyclic drugs)
  Enuresis (imipramine best studied)
  Attention deficit-hyperactivity disorder
  Cataplexy due to narcolepsy
  School phobia and separation anxiety disorder
  Pseudobulbar affect (pathologic laughing and weeping)

Reproduced with permission from Hyman SE, Arana GW, Rosenbaum JF, Handbook of psychiatric drug therapy. 3rd ed. Boston: Little, Brown, and Company, 1995:43.

Panic disorder with or without agoraphobia has been shown to respond to MAOIs, TCAs, and high-potency benzodiazepines (alprazolam and clonazepam). Although not proven, SSRIs seem to have similar clinical efficacy.

Obsessive-compulsive disorder (OCD) has been shown to respond to the tricyclic clomipramine (Anafranil) and to SSRIs at high doses (fluoxetine 60–80 mg/day). Obsessions tend to be more responsive to pharmacotherapy than compulsions. Symptoms of OCD respond more slowly than major depression. Trials of 12 weeks or more are needed before a medication can be ruled a failure for an OCD patient.

The binging and purging behavior of bulimia has been shown to respond to SSRIs, TCAs, and MAOIs in several open and controlled trials. Because SSRIs have the most benign side-effect profile of these medications, they are often the first-line psychopharmacologic treatment.

▶ MECHANISMS OF ACTION

Antidepressants are thought to exert their effects at particular subsets of neuronal synapses throughout the brain. Their major interaction is with the monoamine neurotransmitter systems (norepinephrine and serotonin). Norepinephrine and serotonin are released throughout the brain by neurons that originate in the locus coeruleus and the raphe nucleus, respectively. These neurotransmitters interact with numerous receptor subtypes in the brain that are associated with the regulation of global state functions including appetite, mood states, arousal, vigilance, attention, and sensory processing.

SSRIs act by binding to presynaptic serotonin reuptake proteins, thereby inhibiting reuptake and increasing the levels of serotonin in the synaptic cleft. TCAs act by blocking presynaptic reuptake of both serotonin and norepinephrine. MAOIs act by inhibiting the presynaptic enzyme (monoamine oxidase) that catabolizes norepinephrine, dopamine, and serotonin, thereby increasing the levels of these neurotransmitters presynaptically.

These immediate mechanisms of action are not sufficient to explain the delayed antidepressant effects (typically 2 to 4 weeks). Other unknown mechanisms must play a role in the successful psychopharmacologic treatment of depression.

▶ CHOICE OF MEDICATION

Because all antidepressants have roughly the same efficacy in treating depression, medication choice is based mainly on symptom profile and diagnosis, prior patient response, and side-effect profile and patient tolerability. SSRIs, bupropion, and venlafaxine are the most well-tolerated antidepressants and are generally thought of as first-line agents for major depression. Compared with TCAs and MAOIs, these medications have very low sedative, anticholinergic, and orthostatic hypotensive effects. The agents should be considered for use especially in patients with cardiac conduction disease, constipation, glaucoma, or prostatic hypertrophy.

Among the tricyclic antidepressants, nortriptyline and desipramine have the least sedative, anticholinergic, and orthostatic hypotensive effects. They can be used as first-line agents in younger healthier people, especially if cost is a consideration (tricyclics are much less expensive than SSRIs, bupropion, or venlafaxine).

Because of the diet restrictions and the risk of postural hypotension, the MAOIs (phenelzine and tranylcypromine) should be used most selectively. They can be quite effective, however, and are used in patients for whom SSRIs and tricyclics have failed, in patients with a concomitant seizure disorder (MAOIs and SSRIs do not lower the seizure threshold), or in those with atypical depressions or social phobia (MAOIs or SSRIs are most effective). High-dose SSRIs and clomipramine (despite its high sedative, anticholinergic, and orthostatic hypotensive effects) are the treatments of choice for OCD.

▶ THERAPEUTIC MONITORING

Approximately 50% of patients who meet DSM-IV criteria for major depression will recover with a single adequate trial (at least 6 weeks at a therapeutic dosage) of an antidepressant. The most common reasons for failed trials are inadequate dose and inadequate trial length. However, dosage and length of trial are often limited by side effects (or noncompliance).

✳ Patients on antidepressants should be monitored carefully for side effects or adverse drug reactions (listed below). Generally, antidepressant therapy of a first episode of unipolar depression should continue for 6 months. Patients with recurrent or chronic depression require longer or perhaps lifelong maintenance treatment. Increasing the dose, augmentation with lithium or T3 (Cytomel), substitution of antidepressants, or addition of a second antidepressant are helpful in treating refractory depression. Patients on most TCAs require serum level measurements to determine appropriate dosing.

▶ SIDE EFFECTS AND ADVERSE DRUG REACTIONS

SSRIs (Fluoxetine, Sertraline, Paroxetine, Fluvoxamine)

Although specific SSRIs have slightly different side-effect profiles, as a group their main side effects are nausea, headache, neuromuscular restlessness (resembling akathisia), insomnia or sedation, and delayed ejaculation/anorgasmia. SSRIs should never be combined with MAOIs: serotonin syndrome may result.

TCAs

Tricyclics in many patients are quite well tolerated but overall are less tolerated by patients for their side effects than the SSRIs, bupropion, or venlafaxine. The major side effects associated with tricyclics are orthostatic hypotension, anticholinergic effects, cardiac toxicity, and sexual dysfunction. Specific TCAs have relative degrees of each of these effects.

Orthostatic hypotension is the most common serious side effect of the TCAs. This is particularly worrisome in elderly patients, who may be more prone to falls.

Anticholinergic toxicity can be mild, including dry mouth, constipation, blurred near vision, and urinary hesitancy, or more severe, with agitation, motor restlessness, hallucinations, delirium, and seizures.

Cardiac toxicity may limit the use of TCAs in some patients. TCAs have quinidine-like effects on the heart, potentially causing sinus tachycardia; supraventricular tachyarrhythmias; ventricular tachycardia; ventricular fibrillation; prolongation of PR, QRS, and QT intervals; bundle branch block; first-, second-, and third-degree heart block; or ST and T-wave changes. Major complications from TCAs are rare in patients with normal hearts. TCAs should be avoided in patients with conduction system disease.

Sexual dysfunction includes impotence in men and decreased sexual arousal in women.

MAOIs

Patients who take MAOIs are at risk for hyperadrenergic crises from the ingestion of sympathomimetic amines (such as tyramine) that fail to be detoxified because of inhibition of the gastrointestinal monoamine oxidase system. Improper diet can lead to severe hypertensive crises (tyramine crisis) with potential myocardial infarction or stroke. Hypertensive crises are a medical emergency. Foods that must be avoided include cured meats or fish, beer, red wine, all cheese except cottage and cream cheeses, and overripe fruits. Many over-the-counter cold and pain remedies must be avoided as well.

MAOIs cause a dose-related orthostatic hypotension: tranylcypromine can cause insomnia and agitation; phenelzine can cause daytime somnolence.

Other Antidepressants

Trazadone is often prescribed as an adjunct to an SSRI for sleep because it has strong sedative properties (at higher doses it serves as an antidepressant). In addition to sedation, trazadone can induce priapism (prolonged, painful, penile erection) that can cause permanent damage. Patients must be instructed to seek emergency treatment should such an erection occur.

Bupropion has a higher than average risk of seizures compared with other antidepressants. The risk of seizures is greatest above a daily dose of 450 mg or after a single dose of greater than 150 mg. *Don't give to Bulimic, Emetic pts.*

Key Points

Antidepressants

1. Antidepressants have multiple indications including various forms of depression, anxiety disorders, bulimia, and obsessive-compulsive disorder, among others.

2. Antidepressants act on serotonergic and noradrenergic receptor systems.

3. Some antidepressants have been shown to be efficacious for particular disorders; however, for major depression, all antidepressants are equally effective and are chosen based on side effect profile and symptom constellation.

4. Some antidepressants, particularly TCAs, require monitoring of serum levels.

5. The effects of antidepressants can be augmented by the addition of lithium or thyroid hormone.

6. Antidepressants have side effects that vary according to class.

CHAPTER 13

Mood Stabilizers

$\mathcal{M}$ood stabilizers are effective in the treatment and prevention of mania, and lithium is also effective in the prophylaxis of **bipolar depression.** In addition, mood stabilizers are used for some forms of nonbipolar impulse control disorders. The mood stabilizers most commonly used are lithium, valproate, and carbamazepine. Valproate and carbamazepine are widely used in neurology, primarily as anticonvulsants. Other medications, such as calcium channel blockers, benzodiazepines, and antipsychotics, have some utility in refractory bipolar disorder.

▶ INDICATIONS

Mood stabilizers are indicated acutely (in conjunction with antipsychotics) for the treatment of mania. They are indicated for long-term maintenance prophylaxis against depression and mania in bipolar individuals. Antiseizure medications (valproate and carbamazepine) also may be useful in individuals having seizure-related mood instability. Mood stabilizers also are used for treatment of impulsive behavior in individuals without bipolar disorders.

The mechanism of action of mood stabilizers in bipolar illness is unclear. The range of neurotransmitters affected by these medications and their disparate modes of action suggests that mania may be controlled by altering the function of several different neurotransmitter systems. Conversely, they may share a common mechanism of action that is yet to be elucidated.

▶ LITHIUM

Mechanism of Action

The mechanism of action of lithium in the treatment of mania is **not well determined.** Lithium alters at least two intracellular second messenger systems (the adenyl cyclase, cyclic AMP system, and the G protein coupled phosphoinositide systems) and as an ion can directly alter ion channel function. Because norepinephrine and serotonin in the central nervous system (CNS) use G protein coupled receptors as one of their mechanisms of action, their function is altered by lithium. Lithium also alters GABA metabolism.

Choice

The choice of mood stabilizer is based on a patient's particular psychiatric illness (i.e., subtype of bipolar disorder) and other clinical factors such as side effects, metabolic routes, patient tolerance, and a history of patient or first-degree relative drug responsiveness. Table 13-1 lists the major mood stabilizers and their most common indications.

Lithium is indicated as a first-line treatment for regular cycling bipolar disorder in individuals with normal renal function. Lithium also is used to augment other antidepressants in unipolar depression. Lithium is renally cleared and can easily reach toxic levels in persons with altered renal function (e.g., especially the elderly). It is less effective in the treatment of the rapid cycling variant of bipolar disorder.

Therapeutic Monitoring

Lithium levels should be monitored regularly until a stable dosing regimen has been obtained. Additional monitoring is necessary in a patient with variable compliance or altered renal function. In addition, patients should be warned about toxicity and be regularly assessed for side effects. Thyroid-stimulating hormone and creatinine should also be monitored at regular intervals to monitor thyroid and kidney function, respectively.

TABLE 13-1	
Psychiatric Indications for Mood Stabilizers	
Drug	Indications
Lithium	Acute mania
0.5-1.2	Long-term prophylaxis in bipolar disorder
	Augmentation of antidepressant medications
	Impulse dyscontrol
Valproate	Acute mania
	Rapid cycling bipolar disorder
	Mixed features bipolar disorder
	Impulse dyscontrol
Carbamazepine	Acute mania
	Rapid cycling bipolar disorder
	Mixed features bipolar disorder
	Impulse dyscontrol

Side Effects

Some common side effects and more serious side effects of mood stabilizers are listed in Table 13-2. Lithium has several minor but troublesome side effects, including tremor, polyuria, gastrointestinal distress, minor memory problems, acne exacerbation, and weight gain. At toxic levels, ataxia, coarse tremor, confusion, coma, sinus arrest, and death can occur. Lithium has a narrow therapeutic window, and patients can become toxic at prescribed doses, especially if they undergo an abrupt change in renal function.

▶ VALPROATE

Mechanism of Action

The mechanism of action of valproate is likely to be its augmentation of GABA function in the CNS. Valproate

---

TABLE 13-2

Drugs Used as Mood Stabilizers

Drug	Side-Effect Profile	
Lithium	Therapeutic levels	
	CNS:	sedation, cognitive clouding, fine tremor
	Endocrine:	abnormal TSH, clinical hypothyroidism
	Cardiac:	T-wave change, sinus arrhythmia
	Renal:	polyuria
	Dermatologic:	acne, psoriasis
	GI:	nausea, vomiting, diarrhea
	Hematologic:	benign leukocytosis
	Other:	weight gain, fluid retention
	Toxic levels	
	CNS:	ataxia, coarse tremor, confusion, seizure, coma, death
	Cardiac:	sinus arrest
Valproate	Therapeutic levels	
	CNS:	somnolence, ataxia, tremor
	Endocrine:	menstrual irregularities, thyroid abnormalities
	Dermatologic:	alopecia, rash
	Hepatic:	mild transaminitis
	GI:	nausea, vomiting, indigestion
	Hematologic:	thrombocytopenia, platelet dysfunction
	Other:	edema
	Toxic levels	
	CNS:	ataxia, confusion, coma, death
	Cardiac:	cardiac arrest
	Idiosyncratic	
	Hepatic:	fatal hepatotoxicity
	GI:	pancreatitis
	Hematologic:	agranulocytosis
Carbamazepine	Therapeutic levels	
	CNS:	ataxia, sedation, dizziness, diplopia
	Dermatologic:	rash
	Cardiac:	decreased atrioventricular conduction
	Hematologic:	benign leukopenia
	GI:	nausea
	Toxic levels	
	CNS:	somnolence, autonomic instability, coma
	Cardiac:	atrioventricular block
	Respiratory:	respiratory depression
	Idiosyncratic	
	Hematologic:	agranulocytosis, pancytopenia, aplastic anemia

Handwritten margin notes: "TSH levels", "Creatinine" (next to Lithium); "Liver Function" (next to Valproate)

Reprinted by permission from Handbook of psychiatric drug therapy. 3rd ed. Hyman SE, Arana GW, Rosenbaum JF, Antipsychotic drugs. Boston: Little, Brown and Company, 1991:127 and 138.

increases GABA synthesis, decreases GABA breakdown, and enhances its postsynaptic efficacy.

Choice

Valproate is indicated in acute mania and in prophylaxis against mania in bipolar disorder (Table 13-1). It is more effective than lithium for the rapid cycling and mixed variants of bipolar disorder. It may not provide prophylaxis against depression in bipolar disorder nor augment antidepressants. It is used in treating impulse dyscontrol.

Therapeutic Monitoring

Valproate levels should be monitored regularly until a stable blood level and dosing regimen has been obtained. Liver function tests should be checked at baseline and frequently during the first 6 months, especially because the idiosyncratic reaction of fatal hepatotoxicity is most frequent in this time frame.

Side Effects

At therapeutic levels, valproate produces a variety of side effects, including sedation, mild tremor, mild ataxia, and gastrointestinal distress. Thrombocytopenia and impaired platelet function may also occur. At toxic levels, confusion, coma, cardiac arrest, and death can occur. Valproate usage carries with it the risk of idiosyncratic but serious side effects. These include fatal hepatotoxicity, fulminant pancreatitis, and agranulocytosis.

▶ CARBAMAZEPINE

Mechanism of Action

The mechanism of action of carbamazepine in bipolar illness is unknown. Carbamazepine alters sodium channel behavior by blocking sodium channels in a use-dependent manner (i.e., carbamazepine alters sodium channels in neurons that have just produced an action potential, blocking the neuron from repetitive firing). In addition, carbamazepine decreases the amount of transmitter release at presynaptic terminals. Carbamazepine also appears to indirectly alter central GABA receptors.

Choice

Carbamazepine is generally considered to be a second-line drug (after lithium and valproate) for the treatment of mania (Table 13-1). It is used in acute mania, prophylaxis against mania in bipolar disorder, and may be more effective than lithium in rapid cycling and mixed mania. Carbamazepine's efficacy in the prophylaxis and treatment of depression is not clear. It is also used in treating impulse dyscontrol.

Side Effects

Carbamazepine, at therapeutic levels, produces similar CNS side effects to lithium and valproate. Nausea, rash, and mild leukopenia also are common. At toxic levels, autonomic instability, atrioventricular block, respiratory depression, and coma can occur. Carbamazepine has idiosyncratic side effects of agranulocytosis, pancytopenia, and aplastic anemia.

Therapeutic Monitoring

Carbamazepine levels should be monitored regularly until a stable dosing regimen has been obtained. Patients should be carefully monitored for rash, signs of toxicity, or evidence of severe bone marrow suppression.

▶ KEY POINTS

Mood stabilizers

1. Are indicated for the treatment of bipolar disorder;
2. Work by unknown but likely varied mechanisms;
3. Have varying efficacy according to the subtype of bipolar illness;
4. Have serious toxicities that require regular monitoring.

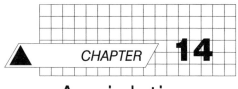

Anxiolytics

$\mathcal{T}$he medications discussed in this chapter have anxiolysis in common. Although benzodiazepines have a wide variety of clinical applications (e.g., as pre-anesthetics, in the treatment of status epilepticus, as muscle relaxants, and in the treatment of insomnia) and other medications (e.g., antidepressants) are of utility in treating some forms of anxiety, the benzodiazepines are uniquely effective for the rapid relief of a broad spectrum of anxiety symptoms. Buspirone is a novel medication that, at present, is used primarily in the treatment of generalized anxiety disorder; it does not appear to be effective in treating other types of anxiety (e.g., panic).

▶ INDICATIONS

Benzodiazepines

Benzodiazepines are among the most widely used drugs in all of medicine. In psychiatry they are used as the primary treatment of a disorder or as adjunct treatment to other pharmacologic agents. Benzodiazepines are used to treat a variety of anxiety disorders: panic disorder, generalized anxiety disorder, anxiety associated with stressful life events (as in adjustment disorders with anxiety), and anxiety that complicates depression (see Chapter 3). In addition, benzodiazepines are used for the short-term treatment of insomnia, for the treatment of alcohol withdrawal, for the agitation of mania, dementia, and psychotic disorders and in the treatment of catatonia (Table 14-1).

Buspirone (Buspar)

Buspirone is used primarily for generalized anxiety disorder.

▶ MECHANISM OF ACTION

Benzodiazepines

Benzodiazepines appear to function as anxiolytics via their agonist action at the central nervous system (CNS) $GABA_A$ receptors (the $GABA_A$ receptor complex regulates a chloride ion channel, $GABA_B$ receptors appear to work by second messenger systems). GABA is a widespread inhibitory neurotransmitter with a complicated receptor structure, having multiple binding sites for GABA, benzodiazepines, and barbiturates. The most likely mode of action of benzodiazepines in treating psychiatric illnesses is via their augmentation of GABA function in the limbic system. Because benzodiazepines are direct agonists at a rapidly responding ion channel, their mechanism of action is virtually instantaneous with their arrival in the CNS (in contrast to buspirone, see below).

Buspirone

Buspirone is a novel medication that appears to act as an anxiolytic via its action as an agonist at the serotonergic $5HT_{1\alpha}$ receptor. In addition, it has some D_2 antagonist effects, although with unclear clinical significance. Unlike the benzodiazepines, it does not work rapidly, but a period of several weeks of sustained dosing is required to exert its symptomatic relief. Buspirone has no GABA receptor affinity and is therefore of no utility in treating benzodiazepine or alcohol withdrawal. Similarly, it is not a sedative and is not useful in treating insomnia.

▶ CHOICE OF MEDICATION

Benzodiazepines

The selection of a benzodiazepine should be based on an understanding of potency, rate of onset, route of

TABLE 14-1

Psychiatric Uses for Benzodiazepines

Anxiety disorders
  Generalized anxiety disorder
  Panic disorder
Mood disorders
  Temporary treatment of anxiety associated with depression
  Temporary treatment of insomnia associated with depression
  Treatment of agitation in acute mania
  Possible mood stabilizing effect in bipolar disorder
Adjustment disorders
  Treatment of adjustment disorder with anxiety
Sleep disorders
  Short-term treatment of insomnia
Miscellaneous
  Treatment of akathisia induced by neuroleptics
  Agitation from psychosis or other causes
  Catatonia (especially lorazepam)
  Alcohol withdrawal

TABLE 14-2
Frequently Used Benzodiazepines

Drug	Oral Dosage Equivalency (mg)*	Onset	Metabolism	Elimination Half-Life†	Active Metab	Common Uses in Psychiatry
Alprazolam (Xanax)	2	Intermediate	Oxidation	6–20	Yes	Panic, anxiety
Chlordiazepoxide (Librium)	40–100	Intermediate	Oxidation	30–100	Yes	Alcohol detoxification
Clonazepam (Klonopin)	1	Intermediate	Oxidation	18–50	No	Panic, anxiety, *Seizures*
Diazepam (Valium)	20	Fast	Oxidation	30–100	Yes	Anxiety, insomnia
Flurazepam (Dalmane)	120	Fast	Oxidation	50–160	Yes	Insomnia
Lorazepam (Ativan)	4	Intermediate	Conjugation	10–20	No	Anxiety, catatonia
Oxazepam (Serax)	60	Slow	Conjugation	8–12	No	Alcohol detoxification
Temazepam (Restoril)	60–120	Intermediate	Conjugation	8–20	No	Insomnia
Triazolam (Halcion)	1	Fast	Oxidation	1.5–5	Yes	Insomnia

*Single dose equivalency.
†In hours. Elimination half-life includes all active metabolites.
Reproduced by permission from Hyman SE, Arana GW, Rosenbaum JF. Handbook of psychiatric drug therapy. 3rd ed. Benzodiazepines and other anxiolytic drugs. Boston: Little, Brown and Company. 1991:151.

metabolism, effective half-life, and clinically proven effectiveness. Although all benzodiazepines appear to function by common mechanisms, the particular combination of the above factors (and perhaps as yet unknown variations in affinity for receptor subtypes) produce varied clinical indications for different benzodiazepines. Table 14-2 illustrates the properties of some commonly used benzodiazepines and their common clinical uses.

Potency   *High = Panic   Xanax, Clonazepam.*
The high-potency benzodiazepines alprazolam and clonazepam are used in the treatment of panic disorder.

Rate of Onset   *Fast = Insomnia.*
Fast-onset benzodiazepines, such as diazepam, may produce a "high" feeling and are potentially more addictive. The fast-onset benzodiazepines flurazepam and triazolam are commonly used for insomnia, as is diazepam.

Route of Metabolism
All benzodiazepines listed, with the exception of lorazepam, oxazepam, and temazepam, require oxidation as a step in their metabolism. Because the oxidative functions of the liver are more vulnerable to liver disease (e.g., cirrhosis) or to a general decline in liver function (e.g., aging), benzodiazepines that require oxidation are more likely to accumulate to toxic levels in individuals with impaired liver function.

Elimination Half-Life
The elimination half-life depicts the effective duration of action of the metabolized medications. For medica-

tions with long elimination half-lives, toxicity easily can occur with repetitive dosing. In addition, toxicology screens may remain positive for several days after the last dose of a long-acting benzodiazepine. Drugs with longer elimination half-lives offer less likelihood of interdose symptom rebound. For example, clonazepam now is favored over alprazolam in the treatment of panic because its longer elimination half-life provides better interdose control of panic symptoms. Medications with shorter elimination half-lives are useful for conditions such as insomnia because they are less likely to produce residual daytime sedation or grogginess.

Active Metabolites
Medications with active metabolites generally have a longer elimination half-life. Among the benzodiazepines, all but three drugs metabolized by conjugation (lorazepam, oxazepam, temazepam) and clonazepam have active metabolites.

Common Uses
Some benzodiazepines are marketed (and more commonly used) for the treatment of a specific disorder (such as alprazolam for panic or triazolam for insomnia).

Buspirone
Buspirone is indicated for the treatment of generalized anxiety disorder. Because of its long lag time to therapeutic effect, patients with severe anxiety symptoms may be unable to sustain a clinical trial. Buspirone is favored as a treatment in individuals with a history of

substance or benzodiazepine abuse. In general, buspirone lacks the reliability of benzodiazepines in relieving anxiety but can be effective in some people.

▶ THERAPEUTIC MONITORING

Benzodiazepines

Benzodiazepine dosing generally is titrated to maximize symptom relief while minimizing side effects and the potential for abuse. No routine monitoring is required; although serum drug levels can be obtained, they are not of great clinical use.

Buspirone

No routine monitoring or drug levels are required when using buspirone.

▶ SIDE EFFECTS AND ADVERSE DRUG REACTIONS

Benzodiazepines

The major side effects of benzodiazepines are related to the CNS. The primary side effect of benzodiazepines is sleepiness or a general groggy feeling. Although benzodiazepines often are used to treat agitation, they may produce disinhibition (and therefore worsen agitation) in some patients. Benzodiazepines are minimally depressive to the respiratory system in healthy individuals but can lead to fatal carbon dioxide retention in patients with chronic obstructive pulmonary disease. In healthy individuals, death after overdose on benzodiazepines alone is rare but does occur when benzodiazepines are taken with alcohol and other CNS depressant medications.

Buspirone

Buspirone does not tend to cause sedation nor does it produce a significant withdrawal syndrome or dependence. The major side effects are dizziness, nervousness, and nausea.

▶ KEY POINTS

Anxiolytics

1. Include benzodiazepines and buspirone;
2. Bind to $GABA_A$ receptors in the cases of benzodiazepines and affect the serotonin receptor in the case of buspirone;
3. Of the benzodiazepine class have a wide variety of uses, including anxiolysis, alcohol detoxification, agitation, and insomnia;
4. Of the benzodiazepine class produce physiologic dependence and may manifest a significant withdrawal syndrome.

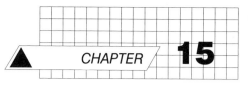

CHAPTER 15

Miscellaneous Medications

*7*his chapter includes medications used commonly in psychiatric practice that do not fall into the conventional categories of psychotherapeutic drugs. Many medications used in general medical practice have side effects such as sedation, stimulation, or anxiolysis. These side effects are often exploited in psychiatry to target specific symptoms (e.g., insomnia, anergia). Other drugs, such as psychostimulants, have precise indications for psychiatric usage. Many more medications than are discussed here are included in the psychiatric armamentarium.

▶ PSYCHOSTIMULANTS

Psychostimulants are used in psychiatry to treat attention deficit disorder, narcolepsy, and some forms of depression (Table 15-1). The most commonly used psychostimulants are dextroamphetamine (Dexedrine), methylphenidate (Ritalin), and pemoline (Cylert). The mechanism of action of these medications appears to occur through their alterations of central nervous system (CNS) monoamine function. Their primary mechanism of action is thought to be facilitating endogenous neurotransmitter release (rather than acting as a direct agonist). Psychostimulants have the liabilities of inducing tolerance and psychological dependence, which may lead to abuse among persons prescribed these medications. The side effects of these medications largely are due to their sympathomimetic actions and include tachycardia, insomnia, anxiety, hypertension, and diaphoresis. Weight loss may be an unwanted side effect (e.g., in young children) but a desirable one in overweight adults.

▶ ANTICHOLINERGICS

Medications with anticholinergic activity are used commonly in psychiatry to treat or provide prophylaxis for some types of neuroleptic-induced movement disorders (Table 15-1). Anticholinergics generally are used as first-line agents in the treatment of neuroleptic-induced parkinsonism and for acute dystonia; they also may have some utility in treating akathisia but are best tried after beta blockers and lorazepam. The most commonly used anticholinergics are benztropine and trihexyphenidyl. In addition, diphenhydramine, an antihistamine that also possesses anticholinergic properties, frequently is used to treat neuroleptic-induced movement disorders and to provide nonspecific sedation. The anticholinergic medications used primarily have CNS antimuscarinic actions. Side effects of anticholinergics due to peripheral anticholinergic action include blurry vision (due to cycloplegia), constipation, and urinary retention; their principal central side effects are sedation and delirium. Anticholinergic toxicity is a major cause of delirium, especially in individuals with dementia and HIV encephalopathy.

▶ BETA BLOCKERS

Beta blockers are used widely in general medicine. In psychiatry, they have a few specific indications (see Table 15-1). Beta blockers likely alter behavior and mood states by altering both central and peripheral catecholamine function. For example, in anxiety, they

TABLE 15-1
Psychiatric Uses of Miscellaneous Medications

Medication	Major Psychiatric Uses
Psychostimulants	Treatment of attention deficit disorder
	Treatment of depression in the elderly or medically ill
	Treatment of narcolepsy
	Augmentation of antidepressants in refractory depression
Anticholinergics *Dystonia/Parkinso.*	Treatment of neuroleptic-induced parkinsonism
	Treatment of neuroleptic-induced dystonia
Beta blockers *Akathesia*	Treatment of impulsivity
	Treatment of some forms of anxiety
	Treatment of akathisia
	Treatment of lithium-induced tremor
Disulfuram	Prevention of alcohol ingestion
Clonidine	Treatment of impulsivity
	Treatment of Gilles de la Tourette syndrome
	Treatment of opiate withdrawal *(sympathetic ↑)*
Tacrine	Treatment of mild to moderate memory loss in Alzheimer's disease
Thyroid hormone	Augmentation of antidepressants in refractory depression

may diminish central arousal; peripherally, they may reduce tachycardia, tremor, sweating, and hyperventilation. Common side effects of beta blockers include bradycardia, hypotension, asthma exacerbation, and masked hypoglycemia in diabetics. Beta blockers also may produce depression-like syndromes characterized by fatigue and depressed mood.

▶ DISULFIRAM (ANTABUSE)

Disulfiram is used to prevent alcohol ingestion through the fear of the consequences of ingesting alcohol while taking disulfiram (Table 15-1). Disulfiram blocks the oxidation of acetaldehyde, a step in the metabolism of alcohol. The buildup of acetaldehyde produces a toxic reaction, making an individual who ingests alcohol while taking disulfiram severely ill. Fatal reactions, although rare, can occur. Disulfiram use should be restricted to carefully selected patients who are highly motivated and who fully understand the consequences of drinking alcohol while taking disulfiram. Side effects in the absence of alcohol ingestion include hepatitis, optic neuritis, and impotence.

▶ CLONIDINE   α2 Agonist - Dec. Sym. Outflow

Clonidine is a CNS alpha$_2$ adrenoreceptor agonist. The alpha$_2$ adrenoreceptor is a presynaptic autoreceptor and inhibits the release of CNS norepinephrine. Clonidine's primary use in medicine is as an antihypertensive (Table 15-1). In psychiatry, clonidine has been variously used. It is effective in decreasing autonomic symptoms associated with opiate withdrawal, in the treatment of Gilles de la Tourette syndrome, and may be useful for impulsiveness and other forms of behavioral dyscontrol. Side effects include sedation, dizziness, and hypotension.

▶ TACRINE   AChE Inh.

Tacrine is an anticholinesterase inhibitor that is used for the treatment of mild to moderate memory loss in Alzheimer's dementia (Table 15-1). Tacrine appears to work by increasing the level of cholinergic function in the cerebral cortex. Initially, treatment with tacrine reduces cognitive impairment; however, this effect wanes with the progressive loss of cholinergic neurons. Tacrine does not alter the course of the disease. Side effects commonly include gastrointestinal upset and cholinomimetic effects, including bradycardia, increased gastric acid secretion, and urinary retention.

▶ THYROID HORMONE   w/ Antidepressants / Li

Thyroid hormones are used primarily in psychiatry to augment the effects of antidepressants (Table 15-1). They also may be used as adjuncts in treating rapid cycling bipolar disorder. Although clinical hypothyroidism can mimic the symptoms of depression, some individuals without clinical hypothyroidism may respond to thyroid augmentation. The theoretic basis for using thyroid hormones lies in the finding of altered hypothalamic-pituitary-adrenal axis functioning in depressed individuals. Although there is debate as to their relative efficacy, both T$_3$ and T$_4$ cross the blood brain barrier. T$_4$ has been shown to be of use in conjunction with lithium to improve clinical control of rapid cycling bipolar disorder. Side effects at low doses are minimal; when dosages result in over-replacement, symptoms of hyperthyroidism emerge.

▶ KEY POINTS

Miscellaneous medications

1. Are widely used for treatment of symptoms and side effects;

2. Overlap with medications used in other medical practice;

3. Have side effects and efficacy specific to each medication and its target symptoms.

CHAPTER 16

Major Adverse Drug Reactions

*7*his chapter describes a group of major adverse reactions associated with use of psychiatric medications. Minor adverse reactions and side effects are outlined in the chapters on respective medications. Although the adverse drug reactions discussed below (with the exception of serotonin syndrome) are most commonly produced by antipsychotic medications, they may occur in response to other medications. The major adverse drug reactions to antipsychotics, their risk factors, onset, and treatment are outlined in Table 16-1. Although the *Diagnostic and Statistical Manual of Mental Disorders*, 4th edition, classifies dystonia, akathisia, extrapyramidal symptoms (EPS), neuroleptic malignant syndrome (NMS), and tardive dyskinesia as neuroleptic-induced movement disorders, it is clear that akathisia can occur with the use of nonneuroleptic psychiatric medications.

▶ DYSTONIA

Dystonia is a neuroleptic-induced movement disorder characterized by muscle spasms. Dystonia commonly involves the musculature of the head and neck but also may include the extremities. Symptoms may range from a mild subjective sensation of increased muscle tension to a life-threatening syndrome of severe muscle tetany and laryngeal dystonia (laryngospasm) with airway compromise. The muscle spasms may lead to abnormal posturing of the head and neck with jaw muscle spasm. Spasm of the tongue leads to macroglossia and dysarthria; pharyngeal dystonia may produce impaired swallowing and drooling. Ocular muscle dystonia may produce oculogyric crisis.

Risk factors include use of high-potency antipsychotics; young men are at increased risk. The condition usually develops early in drug therapy (within days).

TABLE 16-1

Neuroleptic-Induced Movement Disorders*

Disorder	Risk Factors	Onset	Treatment
Dystonia	High-potency antipsychotics →Young men	First few days of therapy	IM/IV benztropine or diphenhydramine Severe laryngospasm may require intubation
Akathisia	Recent increase/onset of medication dosing	First month of therapy	Propanolol, lorazepam, clonidine ?anticholinergics
EPS	High-potency antipsychotics Elderly Prior episode of EPS Mood Disorder.	First few weeks of therapy	Anticholinergic Lower antipsychotic dosage or change to lower potency antipsychotic
NMS	High-dose antipsychotics, rapid dose escalation, or IM injection of antipsychotics Agitation, dehydration Prior episode of NMS	Usually within first few weeks, can occur at any point in antipsychotic therapy	Discontinue antipsychotic medication Supportive symptom management Dantrolene, bromocriptine May require intensive care unit care
Tardive dyskinesia	Elderly Long-term antipsychotic treatment ✗Female gender ✗African-Americans ✗Mood disorders	Usually after years of treatment	Lower dosage of antipsychotic Change antipsychotics Change to clozaril

*The DSM-IV classification for these disorders defines them as neuroleptic-induced movement disorders. The term *neuroleptic* generally refers to typical antipsychotics (see Chapter 11). Exceptions to the term neuroleptic include risperidone, which is classified as an atypical antipsychotic but which can cause all the above disorders; SRIs, which are not neuroleptic drugs but which can clearly produce akathisia; and clozaril, which does not appear to produce dystonia, akathisia, EPS, or tardive dyskinesia but which may cause NMS.

Treatment of dystonia depends on the severity of the symptoms. In the absence of laryngospasm or severe patient discomfort, IM anticholinergic medication (benztropine or diphenhydramine) can be used. In more severe cases or if laryngospasm is present, IV anticholinergic medication is used. Some cases may require intubation if respiratory distress is severe. Discontinuation of the precipitating antipsychotic is sometimes necessary; in other cases, the addition of anticholinergic medications on a standing basis prevents the recurrence of dystonia.

▶ AKATHISIA

Akathisia is a very common side effect produced by antipsychotic medications but also is caused by serotonin reuptake inhibitors. Akathisia consists of a subjective sensation of inner restlessness or a strong desire to move one's body. Individuals with akathisia may appear anxious or agitated. They may pace or move about, unable to sit still. Akathisia can produce severe dysphoria and anxiety in patients and may drive them to become assaultive or to attempt suicide. It is important to accurately diagnose akathisia because if mistaken for agitation or worsening psychosis, antipsychotic dosage may be increased with resultant worsening of the akathisia.

Risk factors for akathisia include a recent increase in medication dosing or the recent onset of medication use. Most cases occur within the first month of drug therapy but can occur anytime during treatment.

Treatment is either with beta blockers (propanolol is commonly used) or benzodiazepines (especially lorazepam). Although there is some doubt as to their efficacy, anticholinergics also are used frequently.

▶ EXTRAPYRAMIDAL SYMPTOMS

EPSs, also known as neuroleptic-induced parkinsonism, consist of the development of the classic symptoms of parkinsonism but in response to neuroleptic use. The most common symptoms are rigidity and akinesia, which occur in as many as half of all patients receiving long-term neuroleptic therapy. A 3- to 6-Hz tremor may be present in the head and face muscles or the limbs. Akinesia or bradykinesia are manifested by decreased spontaneous movement and may be accompanied by drooling. Rigidity consists of the classic parkinsonian "lead pipe" rigidity (rigidity that is present continuously throughout the passive range of motion of an extremity) or cogwheel rigidity (rigidity with a catch and release character).

Risk factors for the development of EPS include the use of high-potency neuroleptics, increasing age, and a prior episode of EPS. EPS usually develop within the first few weeks of therapy.

Treatment consists of reducing the dosage of antipsychotic (if possible) and adding anticholinergic medications to the regimen.

▶ NEUROLEPTIC MALIGNANT SYNDROME

NMS is an idiosyncratic and potentially life-threatening complication of antipsychotic drug use. Symptoms of NMS may develop gradually over a period of hours to days and can often overlap with symptoms of general medical illness. The major clinical findings in patients with NMS are presented in Table 16-2. Many symptoms of NMS are nonspecific and overlap with symptoms common to other psychiatric and medical conditions. The diagnosis of NMS also is complicated by the waxing and waning nature of the clinical picture. As a result, the diagnosis of NMS often is very difficult.

Autonomic instability coupled with motor abnormalities are essential to the diagnosis of NMS. Autonomic alterations can include cardiovascular alterations with cardiac arrhythmias and labile blood pressure. Low-grade fever progressing to severe hyperthermia also may be present. Motor findings may overlap with other motor abnormalities in psychiatric illness, for example, rigidity/dystonia can be confused

---

TABLE 16-2

Neuroleptic Malignant Syndrome

Autonomic
  Tachycardia, other cardiac arrhythmias
  Hypertension
  Hypotension
  Diaphoresis
  Fever progressing to hyperthermia
Motor
  Rigidity/dystonia
  Akinesia
  Mutism
  Dysphagia
Behavioral
  Agitation
  Incontinence
  Delirium
  Seizures
  Coma
Laboratory
  Increased creatine kinase
  Abnormal liver function tests
  Increased white blood cell count

with simple dystonia or with EPS. Mutism can be a sign of severe psychosis or catatonia alone, although this does occur with NMS. Behavioral features such as agitation can also overlap with other psychiatric syndromes; however, the presence of delirium or seizures are harbingers of more serious general medical illness (including drug withdrawal) or NMS. Laboratory findings may reveal an increased creatine kinase secondary to myonecrosis from sustained muscular rigidity. Liver enzymes may be elevated, but their relation to NMS is unclear. Leukocytosis is also often present.

Risk factors for the development of NMS (see Table 16-1) include the use of high-dose antipsychotics, rapid dose escalation, IM injection of antipsychotics, dehydration, agitation, or a prior history of NMS. Some factors may be related to severity of illness (e.g., severely ill patients often have poor oral intake and become dehydrated, are more likely to be placed in restraints, and require IM injection of an antipsychotic) rather than causative factors. Although NMS is most common during the first few weeks of antipsychotic drug therapy, it can occur at any time during therapy.

Treatment of this potentially fatal disorder is largely supportive. Specific interventions include discontinuation of antipsychotics (an option that may take a long period of time in individuals treated with depot antipsychotics); dantrolene (a muscle relaxant) is used to treat rigidity and decrease myonecrosis and bromocriptine (a dopamine agonist) sometimes is used to reverse dopamine blocking effects of antipsychotics. Symptom management including intensive care unit level of care with cardiac monitoring and

intubation may be necessary. Symptoms of NMS overlap with the serotonin syndrome (Table 16-3). However, in NMS, muscular rigidity and increased creatine kinase are prominent findings. In addition, serotonin syndrome develops in response to use of multiple medications that affect serotonin function (especially monoamine oxidase inhibitors [MAOIs]), whereas NMS develops in response to antipsychotic medications. In patients where both MAOIs and antipsychotics are used (e.g., refractory psychotic depression), the differential diagnosis can be quite difficult.

▶ TARDIVE DYSKINESIA

Tardive dyskinesia (TD) is a movement disorder that develops with long-term neuroleptic use; rarely, especially in the elderly, onset may not be as delayed. TD consists of constant, involuntary, stereotyped choreoathetoid movements most frequently confined to the head and neck musculature but also involving, at times, the extremities and respiratory and oropharyngeal musculature.

Risk factors include long-term treatment with neuroleptics, increasing age, female sex, and the presence of a mood disorder. Although TD is reversible in some cases, it tends to be permanent.

Treatment consists of changing antipsychotics, lowering their dosage, or switching to clozapine. Clozapine, which appears to work by a different mechanism from other antipsychotics, may reduce or eliminate the abnormal movements in TD.

▶ SEROTONIN SYNDROME *MAOI'S +*

Serotonin syndrome can occur when multiple medications are used that alter serotonin metabolism. Classically, this syndrome is produced when other serotonin-altering medications are used with MAOIs. This syndrome, which can be life threatening, consists of symptoms outlined in Table 16-3. These include severe autonomic instability, motor abnormalities, and behavioral changes. The course of the disorder can become malignant and end in coma and death. A similar syndrome can be produced when MAOIs are used with meperidine or dextromethorphan and perhaps other opiates.

Serotonin syndrome has many similarities to NMS. The major diagnostic differentiation is based on the absence of increased muscular rigidity and dystonic syndromes in serotonin syndrome and the fact that it is precipitated by the use of MAOIs with other serotonin-altering agents. NMS is precipitated by the use of antipsychotics.

TABLE 16-3

Serotonin Syndrome

Autonomic
 Tachycardia
 Hypertension
 Diaphoresis
 Fever progressing to hyperthermia
Motor
 Shivering
 Myoclonus
 Tremor
 Hyperreflexia
 Oculomotor abnormalities
Behavioral
 Restlessness
 Agitation
 Delirium
 Coma

Risk factors for serotonin syndrome, other than combining MAOIs with other serotonin-altering medications, are not known.

Treatment for serotonin syndrome is largely supportive and may require intensive care unit level of care with cardiac monitoring and intubation. The offending medications should be discontinued.

▶ **KEY POINTS**

Major adverse drug reactions

1. Occur most commonly in psychiatry with use of antipsychotics and serotonin altering medications;

2. Consist of dystonia, akathisia, EPS, NMS, and TD in the case of antipsychotics;

3. Consist of akathisia and the serotonin syndrome in the case of serotonin altering medications;

4. Are largely reversible with the exception of TD, which may be permanent.

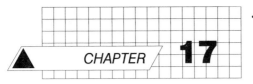
Psychological Theories

*T*here are a large number of competing theories influencing contemporary psychotherapeutic thinking. Psychotherapies derived from psychoanalytic, cognitive, and behavior theory are the most widely used. Cognitive and behavioral interventions have the greatest empirical verification.

▶ PSYCHOANALYTIC/PSYCHODYNAMIC THEORY

The principal theorist responsible for launching psychoanalysis as a technique and psychodynamic theory in general is Sigmund Freud. Freud's theories proposed that unconscious motivations and early developmental influences were essential to understanding behavior. Freud's original theories have proven quite controversial and have led to the creation of various alternative or derivative theories.

Twentieth Century Schools of Psychodynamic Psychology

There are three major twentieth century psychodynamic schools: Drive Psychology, Ego Psychology, and Object Relations Theory.

Drive Psychology

Drive psychology posited that infants have sexual (and other) drives. This theory proposed that sexual and aggressive instincts are present in each individual and that each individual passes sequentially through psychosexual developmental stages (named oral, anal, phallic, and genital). Included in drive psychology is conflict theory, which proposes to explain how character and personality development are influenced by the interaction of drives with the conscience and reality.

Ego Psychology

Freud eventually developed a tripartite theory of the mind in which the psychic structure was composed of the id, ego, and superego. Under this theory, the id was the compartment of the mind containing the drives and instincts. The superego contained the sense of right and wrong, largely derived from parental and societal morality. The ego was responsible for adaptation to the environment and for the resolution of conflict. A major function of the ego was the reduction of anxiety. Ego defenses (Table 17-1) were proposed as psychic mechanisms that protected the ego from anxiety. Some ego defenses (e.g., sublimation) are more functional to the individual than others (e.g., denial).

Object Relations Theory

Object relations theory (*objects* refers to important people in one's life) departed from drive theory in that the relationship to an object was motivated by the primacy of the relationship rather than the object being a means of satisfying a drive. Child observation furthered object relations theory, emphasizing concepts of attachment and separation.

TABLE 17-1

Common Ego Defense Mechanisms

Denial	Feelings or ideas that are distressing to the ego are blocked by refusing to recognize evidence for their existence.
Projection	Feelings or ideas that are distressing to the ego are attributed to others.
Regression	Feelings or ideas that are distressing to the ego are reduced by behavioral return to an earlier development phase.
Repression	Feelings or ideas that are distressing to the ego are relegated to the unconscious.
Reaction formation	Feelings or ideas that are distressing to the ego are converted into their opposites.
Displacement	Feelings or ideas that are distressing to the ego are redirected to a substitute that evokes a less intense emotional response.
Rationalization	Feelings or ideas that are distressing to the ego are dealt with by creating an acceptable alternative explanation.
Suppression	Feelings or ideas that are distressing to the ego are not dealt with but they remain components of conscious awareness.
Sublimation	Feelings or ideas that are distressing to the ego are converted to those that are more acceptable.

The interpersonal school arose as an outgrowth of object relations theory. The interpersonal theorists emphasized that intrapsychic conflicts are less important than one's relationship to one's sense of self and to others. In other words, the relationships in a person's life are given primary importance in producing happiness or misery.

► ERIKSON'S LIFE CYCLE THEORY

Erik Erikson made major contributions to the concept of ego development. Erikson theorized that ego development persisted throughout one's life. Erikson conceptualized that psychosocial events drive change, leading to a developmental crisis. Under Erikson's model, individuals passed through a series of life cycle stages (Table 17-2). Each stage presented core conflicts produced by the interaction of developmental possibility with the external world. Individual progress and associated ego development occurred with successful resolution of the developmental crisis inherent in each stage. This model allowed for continued ego development until death.

► COGNITIVE THEORY

Cognitive theory recognizes the importance of the subjective experience of oneself, others, and the world. It posits that irrational beliefs and thoughts about oneself, the world, and one's future can lead to psychopathology.

In cognitive theory, thoughts or cognitions regarding an experience determine the emotions that are evoked by the experience. For example, the perception of danger in a situation naturally leads to anxiety. When danger is truly present, anxiety can be adaptive, leading to hypervigilance and self-protection. When the situation is only perceived as dangerous (such as in fear of public speaking), the resulting anxiety can be psychologically paralyzing. The person may fear public speaking because of an irrational fear that something disastrous will occur in public. A principal type of irrational belief is a cognitive distortion (Table 17-3).

► BEHAVIORAL THEORY

Behavioral theory posits that behaviors are fashioned through various forms of learning, including modeling, classic conditioning, and operant conditioning (Table 17-4). A behaviorist might propose that through operant conditioning, depression is caused by a lack of

---

TABLE 17-2

Erikson's Life Cycle Stages

Trust versus mistrust	Birth to 18 mo	The infant has many needs but does not have the power to have those needs met. The child is dependent on caretakers. If caretaking is appropriate, a sense of trust and hope are created. If inappropriate or inadequate, mistrust develops.
Autonomy versus shame	18 mo to 3 yr	The child is learning about the use of language and control of bowel and bladder function and walking. As a result, it begins to choose to influence and explore the world. If caretaking is appropriate, the child will develop a healthy balance between exerting its autonomy and feeling shame over the consequences of exerting autonomy.
Initiative versus guilt	3–5 yr	As the child develops increasing control of language and walking, he or she has increased initiative to explore the world. The potential for action carries with it the risk of guilt at indulging forbidden wishes.
Industry versus inferiority	5–13 yr	The child begins to develop a sense of self based on the things it creates. Caretaker influences are important in helping the child develop a sense of mastery and competence over creating.
Industry versus identity confusion	13–21 yr	Corresponds to adolescence. How one appears to others is important in this stage. There are conflicts between one's identity and the need to gain acceptance.
Intimacy versus isolation	21–40 yr	The anxiety and vulnerability produced by intimacy are balanced against the loneliness produced by isolation.
Generativity versus stagnation	40–60 yr	If successful, the individual develops a positive view of his or her role in life and a sense of commitment to society at large. If unsuccessful, individuals move through life without concern for the greater welfare.
Integrity versus despair	60 yr to death	An individual accepts one's life course as appropriate and necessary. If this fails, the individual may regret or wish to relive some part of life, leading to despair.

TABLE 17-3

Types of Cognitive Distortions

Arbitrary inference	Drawing a specific conclusion without sufficient evidence
Dichotomous thinking	A tendency to categorize experience as "all or none"
Overgeneralization	Forming and applying a general conclusion based on an isolated event
Magnification/ minimization	Overvaluing or undervaluing the significance of a particular event

positive reinforcement (as may occur after the death of a spouse), resulting in a general lack of interest in behaviors that were once pleasurable (or reinforced).

▶ **COGNITIVE-BEHAVIORAL THERAPY**

Cognitive and behavioral theories form part of the bases of cognitive-behavioral therapy (CBT). CBT involves the examination of cognitive distortions and the use of behavioral techniques to treat common disorders such as major depression.

▶ **KEY POINTS**

Psychological theories

1. Are numerous, but those derived from psychoanalytic, cognitive, and behavior theory are most widely used;

2. Derived from the psychoanalytic school emphasize unconscious motivations and early influences;

3. Derived from the cognitive school emphasize subjective experience, beliefs, and thoughts;

4. Derived from the behavioral school emphasize the influence of learning;

5. Derived from the cognitive and behavioral schools have the greatest empiric support.

TABLE 17-4

Important Concepts in Behavior Theory

Modeling	A form of learning based on observing others and imitating their actions and responses
Classic conditioning	A form of learning in which a neutral stimulus is repetitively paired with a natural stimulus, with the result that the previously neutral stimulus alone becomes capable of eliciting the same response as the natural stimulus
Operant conditioning	A form of learning in which environmental events (contingencies) influence the acquisition of new behaviors or the extinction of existing behaviors

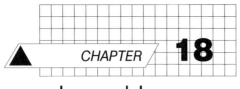

CHAPTER 18

Legal Issues

 Legal issues affect all areas of medicine, particularly psychiatry. The laws that govern medical practice address physician duty, negligence, and malpractice as well as patient competence, consent, and right to refuse treatment. Previous court decisions, or precedents, are used as the standard by which a given action (or inaction) is judged. Practitioners should be aware of the pertinent laws of the state in which they practice to comply adequately with standards of practice while respecting the rights and duties of their role. Reducing adverse events and legal claims in the health care system is known as risk management.

▶ MALPRACTICE

The legal definition of malpractice requires the presence of four elements: negligence, duty, direct causation, and damages. Negligence can be thought of as failure to perform some task with respect to the patient that falls short of the care that would be provided by the average practitioner (the standard of care). Duty reflects the law's recognition of the obligation of the physician to provide proper care to his or her patients. Direct causation requires that the negligence directly caused the alleged damages. Finally, damages (e.g., physical or emotional harm) must in fact be shown to have occurred. In short, malpractice involves the negligence of a duty that directly causes damages. Malpractice claims in psychiatry principally involve suicides of patients in treatment, misdiagnosis, medication complications, false imprisonment (involuntary hospitalization or seclusion), and sexual relations with patients.

▶ INFORMED CONSENT

Informed consent has three components: information, consent, and competence. First, appropriate levels of information regarding a proposed treatment, including side effects, alternative treatments, and outcome without treatment, must be provided. Second, the patient must be competent (i.e., have the capacity to understand, reason, and make reasonable decisions regarding the risks and benefits of treatment). Third, the patient must give consent voluntarily. The patient must not be coerced into giving consent. True emergency situations are an exception to this rule; treatments necessary to stabilize a patient in an emergency can be given without informed consent.

▶ INVOLUNTARY COMMITMENT

Commitments generally are judicially supported actions that require persons to be hospitalized or treated against their will. Although laws vary from state to state, commitment criteria usually require evidence that the patient is a danger to self, danger to others, or is unable to care for him or herself. Psychiatrists, in most localities, have the right to temporarily involuntarily commit a patient if any of these criteria are met, and a diagnosis of a mental disorder is provided (in other words, both a mental disorder and danger must exist). The duration of temporary commitment and the rights of the patient vary by jurisdiction. Patients who have been committed have a right to be treated, and unless they have been declared incompetent, they have the right to refuse treatment.

▶ THE TARASOFF DECISIONS: DUTY TO WARN (OR PROTECT)

Tarasoff *v* The Board of Regents of the University of California (or simply, Tarasoff) was a landmark case that was heard twice in the California Supreme Court in 1976. Tarasoff I held that therapists have a duty to warn the potential victims of their patients. Tarasoff II held that therapists have a duty to take reasonable steps to protect potential victims of their patients. In most localities, this means that the therapist should take reasonable action to protect a third party if a patient has specifically identified the third party and a risk of serious harm seems imminent.

▶ M'NAGHTEN RULE: THE INSANITY DEFENSE

Named after a mentally ill man (M'Naghten) who attempted to assassinate the prime minister of England in 1843, the rule forms the basis of the insanity defense. The gist of the M'Naghten rule is that a person is not held responsible for a criminal act *if* at the time the act was performed, he or she suffered from mental

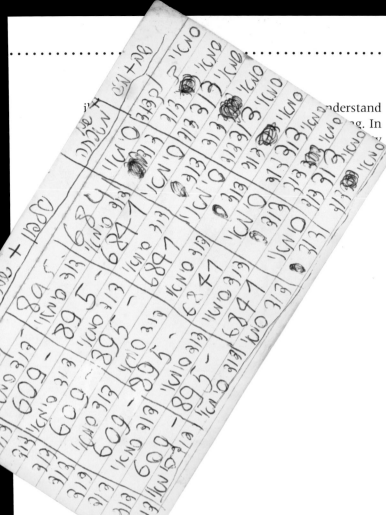

nderstand
g. In

orists argue for the designation "guilty but insane" to indicate culpability but at the same time recognize the presence of a mental illness (and presumably the need for treatment).

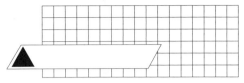

Selected References

Adams D, Victor M. Principles of neurology. 4th ed. New York: McGraw-Hill, Inc., 1989.

Andreasen NC, Black DW. Introductory textbook of psychiatry. 2nd ed. Washington, DC: American Psychiatric Press, Inc., 1995.

Baldessarini RJ. Chemotherapy in psychiatry: principles and practice. Cambridge: Harvard University Press, 1985.

Corsini RJ, Wedding D. Current psychotherapies. 5th ed. Itasca: E. F. Peacock Publishers, Inc., 1995.

Davison GC, Neale JM. Abnormal psychology: an experimental clinical approach. 4th ed. New York: John Wiley & Sons, Inc., 1986.

Diagnostic and statistical manual of mental disorders. 4th ed. Washington, DC: American Psychiatric Association, 1994.

Hyman SE, Arana GW, Rosenbaum JF. Handbook of psychiatric drug therapy. 3rd ed. Boston: Little, Brown and Company, 1991.

Kaplan HI, Sadock BJ. Comprehensive textbook of psychiatry. 6th ed. Baltimore: Williams & Wilkins, 1995.

Index